D1085678

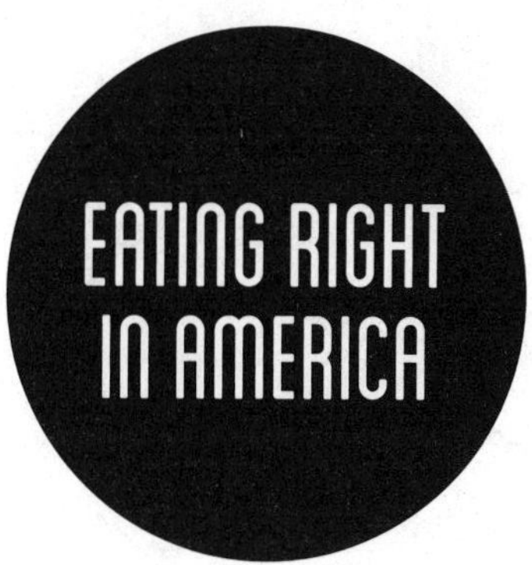

EATING RIGHT
IN AMERICA

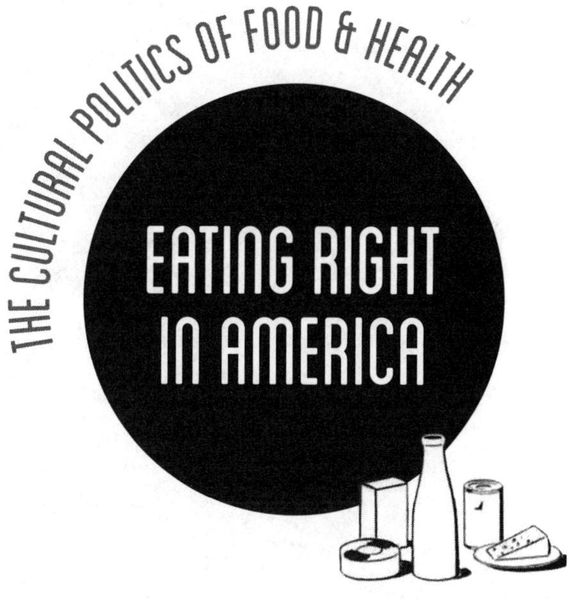

Charlotte Biltekoff

Duke University Press • Durham and London • 2013

 Printed in the United States of America on acid-free paper ∞. Designed by Courtney Leigh Baker and Typeset in Minion Pro with Blanch display by Keystone Typesetting, Inc.

Library of Congress Cataloging-in-Publication Data
Biltekoff, Charlotte.
Eating right in America : the cultural politics of food and health / Charlotte Biltekoff.
pages cm
Includes bibliographical references and index.
ISBN 978-0-8223-5544-1 (cloth : alk. paper)
ISBN 978-0-8223-5559-5 (pbk. : alk. paper)
1. Nutrition—United States. 2. Diet—United States. 3. Food habits—United States. I. Title.
TX360.U6B548 2013
394.1′20973—dc23
2013013823

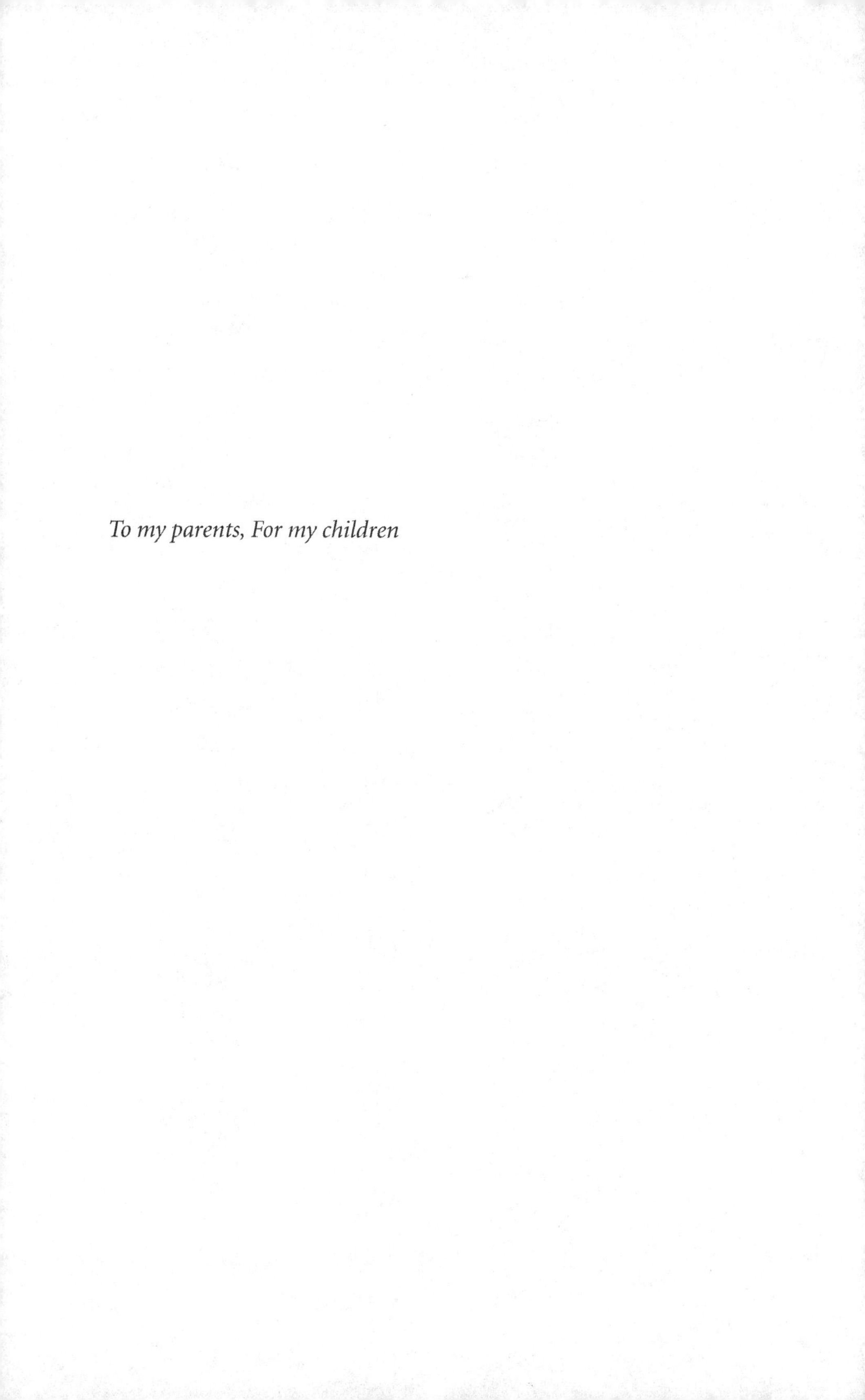

To my parents, For my children

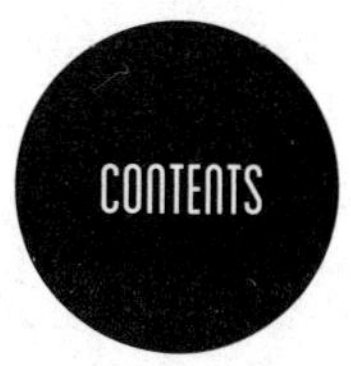
CONTENTS

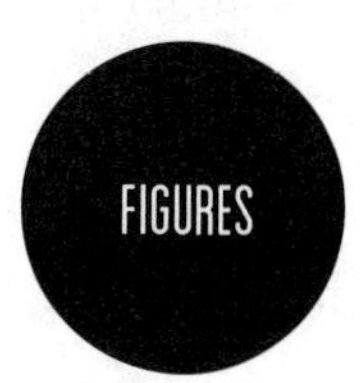

The food problem is fundamental to the welfare of the race. Society, to protect itself, must take cognizance of the question of food and nutrition.
—ELLEN RICHARDS • 1910

Defense is . . . building the health, the physical fitness, the social well-being of all our people, and doing it the democratic way. Hungry people, undernourished people, ill people, do not make for strong defense. —HARRIET ELLIOT • 1940

I believe our destiny as a nation depends on how we nourish ourselves. . . . The way we produce, prepare and eat food expresses the bedrock values on which our public and private lives are built.
—ALICE WATERS • 1992

We are at a crossroads in our nation. We're standing at the corners of health and disease. Are we going to sentence ourselves to being a society defined by obesity and disease? Or are we going to choose to be a nation of health and vitality?
—SURGEON GENERAL RICHARD CARMONA • 2003

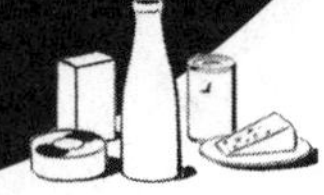

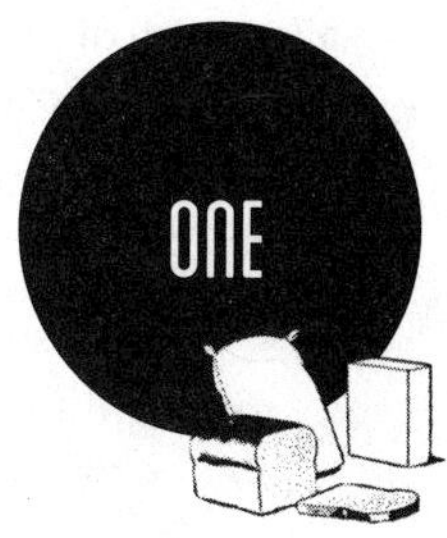

THE CULTURAL POLITICS OF DIETARY HEALTH

This project began in the mid-1990s when I was working as a cook in San Francisco and discovered a book called *Perfection Salad* in a used bookstore.[1] Laura Shapiro's history of the domestic science movement enthralled me both because of the story it told, through food, about the aspirations of a generation of women responding to industrialization, urbanization, and immigration and because its very existence assured me that, as I had suspected, it was possible and productive to rethink American history through the lens of food. Shapiro's subjects were reformers who believed that changing what people ate could improve their morals and character and ultimately could address some of the most difficult social problems—from intemperance to labor unrest—arising in the rapidly industrializing urban centers of the American Northeast. Ellen Richards, the leader of the domestic science movement, was convinced that teaching people to eat right was essential to creating responsible and moral citizens and maintaining a stable social order. I was struck by the resonance between these ideas about the social importance of eating habits one hundred years earlier and what a certain restaurateur-turned-activist was beginning to preach to a very receptive audience in Berkeley and beyond. Alice Waters was passionately urging people to recognize the connection between eating and ethics, and through her Edible Schoolyard project was attempting to show exactly how teaching people to eat right could create responsible citizens and address problems in the social order—from nihilism to violence and environmental degradation.

Waters's ideas about how we should be eating in order to protect our most cherished resources, both social and environmental, resonated with me and many of my friends. I had grown up allergic to milk in the shadow of a family dairy business—my great grandfather had started making cottage cheese in his bathtub in the 1920s, and by the time I came along the business had grown to include yogurt, sour cream, and chip dip—so I knew something about the social significance of eating habits. I learned even more about the politics of dietary choice and the complex relationships between morality and health after, without giving it much thought, I became a vegetarian at the age of thirteen (remaining so for about seventeen years). I barely made it through my second year of college on the East Coast before declaring that I was moving to California to "work with vegetables," and by the time I discovered Shapiro and Waters I was a cook at Greens, a well-known vegetarian restaurant in San Francisco founded in 1979 by the San Francisco Zen Center. In the Greens kitchen I absorbed the meaningfulness of the seasons, learned to express my appreciation of good produce through skilled but restrained technique, and developed a worldview in which food was a language for emotions, relationships, and values. I wrote a food column for a local paper, published a community cookbook called *Delicious*, which was bound with chopsticks and wire, and gave readings at local open mics with a wooden spoon in my pocket. Greens was in many ways a cultural and culinary sibling of Waters's Chez Panisse, and Waters's ideas seemed utterly sensible, intuitive, and right to me. Of course we should eat ethically, value the table as a place for community and family, know where our food came from. But the hundred-year-old voice of Ellen Richards taunted me into questioning, instead of joining, the revolution.

Waters's convictions were surprisingly similar to Richards's. While Waters's aim was to overturn exactly the changes in the food system that Shapiro credits the domestic scientists with ushering in (scientific rationality, standardization, industrialization), she shared Richards's fundamental insistence that teaching people to eat right was essential to social well-being and that, by ignoring food, the public schools were failing in their mandate to train citizens. How could two reformers with such entirely different ideas about how people should eat be at the same time so completely alike in their convictions about *why* it was important to teach people how to eat? Clearly there was something meaningful about telling people how to eat right that transcended the dietary advice itself.

I enrolled in the University of California, Berkeley, to pursue these questions and finish my undergraduate degree. I cut back my hours at Greens, traded creative writing about food for academic writing about food reformers, and wrote a senior thesis called "Banana Salad and Squash Blossoms: A Comparative History of Two Food Reform Movements." The thesis was an exploration of the relationship between the domestic science movement and the "Delicious Revolution" that Alice Waters was fomenting. Through the process of researching and writing, I came to believe that the relationship between Richards and Waters was not at all random or coincidental, but rather the result of a set of cultural beliefs about the meaning of eating right that inspired both of them to see improving people's eating habits as a way to improve their moral character. I began to understand that the reformers involved in both movements played a certain cultural role even when they were not aware of doing so, delineating social norms and imposing the values of the middle class through the seemingly neutral language of diet. My qualms about joining Waters's revolution evolved into a critique of the dietary reform impulse itself, and I started to find it odd that dietary advice was commonly treated as nothing more than the beneficent application of knowledge to the aspiration of living better, healthier lives. By the time national alarm about obesity had reached a near deafening pitch, in the late 1990s, I was in graduate school. Having seen dire warnings about the diets of Americans before—in Ellen Richards's early-twentieth-century caution that the future of the race depended on eating habits, for example—I was certain that understanding the history of dietary reform was essential to making sense of the campaign against obesity and its social ramifications.

While this book is about dietary reform, my aim is not to change people's eating habits. Instead, I hope to illuminate the cultural politics of dietary health in America so we can better understand what happens when we define good diets, talk about eating right, or try to improve other people's eating habits. What are we really talking about when we talk about dietary health? Why is the question of what to eat so morally fraught? Why is teaching people to eat right such a compelling project for the American middle class? What does it really mean to eat right in America? I present the stories of four seemingly distinct reform movements, exposing their continuities and discontinuities, in order to answer these questions. I start with the contention that despite seemingly scientific origins, dietary ideals are cultural, subjective, and political. While its primary aim may be to improve health, the process of teaching people to "eat right" inevitably involves shaping certain kinds of subjects, and citizens, and shoring up the identity and social boundaries of the ever-threatened American middle class.

The story I tell here is about dietary ideals and the people who have dedicated themselves to promoting "eating right" as a biological and social good. While it's designed to help us understand the social role of ideas about "good diets," this story also illuminates several larger issues, including the cultural politics of health, the historical dynamics of class, and the process of social normalization. The history of dietary reform, for example, raises questions about the massive role that health and health promotion has come to play in our individual and social lives over the last century, and particularly since the 1970s. In tracing this expansion through the history of dietary reform, I hope to provoke a dialogue about what health really means to us, and what its pursuit should look like. Are there important social concerns and aims that the emphasis on health obscures rather than promotes? This history also gives us a chance to think anew about how culturally constructed class differences can come to seem like the natural basis for, rather than the result of, social distinction.[2] I hope to cause readers to think about dietary health as a privilege with consequences that extend far beyond the biomedical. The history of dietary reform also adds to our understanding of how ideas about proper behavior and good citizenship are worked out. This history reveals a means of normalization that is usually obscured by the assumed objectivity of scientific discourses, reminding us that in order to understand and act responsibly within the social world we inhabit, we must be bold about the scope of our critical thinking, extending cultural criticism into realms—like dietary health—that are often reserved for science.

On one hand this book is a chronological journey through dietary advice from the late nineteenth century to the present. I take the reader through four distinct dietary reform movements, each one motivated by a unique set of social and nutritional concerns and oriented around its own definitions of what constitutes a good diet and what constitutes a good eater. I start with the domestic science movement at the end of the nineteenth century, move on to the national nutrition program of the World War II home front, then look at two different movements that coalesced toward the end of the twentieth century: the alternative food movement and the campaign against obesity. The chronological narrative focuses both on the ongoing relationship between dietary ideals and social ideals and on the evolving nature of those ideals as they have been reshaped by changes in nutritional knowledge as well as in political, economic, and social pressures. I demonstrate that the scope and purview of dietary reform has grown dramatically over the course of the last century, thus providing a new explanation for why we worry so much about eating right today: not because of an increasing incidence of diet-related diseases or because of growing knowledge about the role of diet in preventing such diseases, but because of ongoing expansions in the social significance of dietary health and the moral valence of being a "good eater."

On the other hand, and on a slightly more abstract level, this book is a conceptual journey from a place where we know exactly what dietary advice is—rules about what to eat based on nutritional findings and aimed at improving health and longevity—to a place of disorientation about what dietary advice is. I want to encourage a rethinking of exactly what it is we think we know about dietary health. In her analysis of the nineteenth-century culture of health, Joan Burbick writes, "Common sense statements in a culture are . . . an index of certain beliefs so dear to the heart of the people that they are presented as the bedrock of reality."[3] While the facts of food and health are certainly the subject of intense debates, the notion that dietary advice is an objective reflection of scientific knowledge and that its primary aim is to produce healthier bodies is "an index of certain beliefs" that I seek to reveal and understand in *Eating Right in America*. The chronological journey through the history of dietary reform is the vehicle for this intellectual journey from what we might call an "empirical" view of dietary health as an objective reflection of nutrition facts to what we might call a "constructionist" view that takes seriously the social and cultural process through which those facts attain their authority and their seeming naturalness.

Two ideas are particularly important to the intertwined historical and theoretical aims of this project. First is that health is fundamentally a cultural concept. The sociologist Robert Crawford describes *health* as a "key word" and highlights the cultural content and the social dynamics of health discourses.[4] Crawford explains, "Talking about health is a way people give expression to our cultural notion of well-being or quality of life. . . . 'Health' provides a means for personal and social evaluation."

Furthermore, he argues, health is a "moral discourse," a means of establishing and affirming shared values around what it is to be a good person.[5] If indeed health is a cultural concept, a means of expressing core cultural values and a moral discourse through which we assess ourselves and others, then dietary health is clearly about more than a physiological relationship between food and the body.

My conversations with students bear out this contention and reveal how cultural values are entwined with our commonsense ideas about eating right. In a course I teach about the culture of food and health in the United States, I begin by asking who in the room tries to eat a "good" or "healthy" diet. Almost all of the students raise their hands. I then ask them to explain *why* they try to "eat right," typically ending up with a blackboard list that reads something like this: to get a date or find a mate (be attractive, be sexy, look hot); to have energy for sports, work, or schoolwork; to obey parents, grandparents or teachers who told me to; to live longer; to avoid disease (because diabetes or heart disease or cancer runs in the family); to show I am educated; to show I am disciplined; to be responsible; because I feel guilty if I do not. The list includes some reasons for eating right that have nothing to do with health (being sexy, displaying discipline, responsibility, or education) and others that appear to be more biomedical, such as seeking energy or longevity and wanting to avoid disease. But even seemingly biomedical motivations for maintaining a good diet are inseparable from cultural values. Aren't efficiency, productivity, and longevity culturally distinct personal goals that have to do with shared cultural values? Is this not also true for the idea that individuals can, and should, mitigate disease through good behavior? The classroom exercise illustrates an important premise of my analysis: there is no such thing as dietary health apart from social ideals and, therefore, dietary ideals are never simply objective reflections of nutritional facts.

The second concept that is foundational to this project builds on the first: dietary ideals always communicate not only rules for how to choose a "good diet," but also guidelines for how to be a good person. This concept draws on John Coveney's argument that nutrition is both an empirical and an ethical system. Coveney explains that nutrition always serves two functions, providing rules about what to eat that also function as a system through which people construct themselves as certain kinds of subjects.[6] This means that dietary advice conveys messages about what to eat that are at the same time lessons in how to be a good eater and a good person. Building on this, my research shows that dietary ideals primarily convey two interlocking sets of social ideals: one communicates emerging cultural notions of good citizenship and prepares people for new social and political realities; the other expresses the social concerns of the middle class and attempts to distinguish its character and identity.

Eating Right in America adds to an emerging body of work that treats nutrition and dietary health as cultural constructs. Histories written by nutrition scientists have, since the emergence of the field itself, approached nutrition as a progressive effort to uncover the truth about food and the human body, tracing the development of scientific methods and discoveries while celebrating their positive impact on human health. Since the 1960s and 1970s social historians have used nutritional data to trace the impact of changes in nutrition status, food supply, and dietary standards on other social conditions, such as the occurrence of deficiency diseases, rates of fertility and mortality, population growth, and worker productivity. Cultural historians influenced by the linguistic turn of the 1970s have treated nutrition as a cultural practice that both shapes and is shaped by other cultural practices, taking into account issues of power, identity, and ideology. Beliefs about the empirical truth of science and the objective reality of the human body that anchor the works described above become the subject of critical inquiry for scholars, like myself, working in an area we might call "critical nutrition studies." We consider nutrition itself—not just its practice but its content—as a product of history. This approach is consistent with poststructuralism's broader impact on the way in which history is viewed and conducted, and it is also shaped by the major insights of science and technology studies about the production of scientific knowledge. My analysis of the history of dietary reform both draws on and seeks to develop two of the key insights that have emerged thus far from this nascent "field": nutrition is not only an empirical set of rules, but also a system of moral measures, and its presumably neutral quantitative strategies are themselves political and ideological.[7]

In approaching dietary health as a cultural concept that conveys social ideals and takes part in the formation of certain kinds of subjects and social formations, I situate *Eating Right in America*, more specifically, at the intersection of the young field of food studies and the even younger field of fat studies. I also illuminate a gap between the two fields that should be developed as a productive intersection. Both food studies and fat studies fall short of providing the full range of tools that we need to critically assess the culture of dietary health in America, but each does provide essential tools for the job. Food studies alerts us to the cultural significance of eating habits and beliefs about food, provides rich insights into the history of those habits and beliefs, and teaches us to be attentive to how power operates through the seemingly mundane. However, in the United States in particular, food studies scholars have taken remarkably little interest in historicizing or theorizing health and have been largely silent on the very important questions that are raised by the distinctly biomedical orientation of American ideas about what is good to eat. The field, therefore, stands to gain much from those scholars engaged in fat studies, in which the body and its social construction are resolutely central.

While fat studies scholarship is acutely aware of the way in which ideas about health are shaped by cultural predispositions and political motivations, its objects of study and its insights are for the most part focused on current and historical manifestations of fatness and its discourses.[8] This is, of course, absolutely essential to building a field that can account for the ways in which fat bodies and subjectivities are constructed, represented, and maligned and how they can be reclaimed. However, such an accounting also requires a broader perspective that investigates the connections between how we think about fat and how we think about food, health, and identity more broadly. An exclusive focus on fat obscures a set of questions that, properly wielded, yield important insights into why the nation is currently mobilized into a war against fat. The campaign against obesity may seem different in kind than a dietary reform movement like domestic science, focusing as it does on body size, rather than on eating habits. But, on the contrary, the antiobesity movement is an extreme manifestation of the logic of dietary reform that emerged at the end of the nineteenth century and an extension of the many expansions in the social role of dietary health that have since occurred.

I begin this history at the end of the nineteenth century because the modern science of human nutrition, which emerged at that time, produced a unique social potential for discourses of eating right. Dietary reformers have helped people to choose diets in accordance with religious or civic ideals since ancient times, and there is an especially interesting and important history of American dietary reformers in the Jacksonian era.[9] There is, however, something unique about the kind of cultural work that dietary reform performs in relation to the seemingly objective, quantitative strategies of science. The phenomenon that I refer to as "modern dietary reform" was born not only because science made it possible to define a "good diet" in empirical terms, but also because the cultural context meant that such a definition was taken as a neutral and authoritative kind of truth. The science of nutrition began its reign as the dominant means of evaluating and categorizing food just as science itself began to secure its cultural status as an arbiter of truth (becoming only more autonomous and seemingly objective over the course of the twentieth century).[10] Therefore, since the late nineteenth century the ethical content of nutrition has been increasingly obscured even as it has been consistently embraced by reformers who undertake the process of dietary improvement in order to achieve social aims, such as the building of character and the melioration of various forms of social instability. The marriage of scientific empiricism with the social aims of dietary reformers defined a new era in which quantifiable norms provided a seemingly objective but nonetheless moral measure of "eating right."

In each chapter of this book I focus on one reform movement and follow roughly the same trajectory, first tracing the emergence of new dietary ideals in relation to both nutritional and social concerns; then examining the relationship between the new dietary ideals and emerging cultural notions of citizenship to show how lessons in eating right have also functioned as a pedagogy of good citizenship; and finally exploring the dynamics of class that are implicated in each discourse of eating right. After I introduce the era of modern dietary reform, the narrative highlights a series of expansions in the role of dietary reform and the social valence of eating right over the last century, helping to explain why questions about what to eat are so pervasive, and fraught, today.

In chapter 2 I focus on the emergence of the era of modern dietary reform and establish an understanding of nutrition as both empirical and ethical. I explore how domestic scientists capitalized on both of these aspects in their promotion of scientific cookery first among the urban poor and later among the "intelligent classes," and argue that courses in home economics taught more than just domestic skills; they helped students to understand and meet the changing demands of citizenship in the context of Progressive Era social and political reforms. I also argue that domestic scientists played a role in forging a distinct middle-class identity in relation to health and introduce the concept of the "unhealthy other," a dynamic through which the middle class affirms its status through the ongoing production of an other whose dangerous diets threaten social stability.[11]

I open chapter 3 by looking at the changes in nutritional thinking brought about by the discovery of vitamins and explore how anxieties and aspirations about the eating habits of the population converged with social concerns related to mobilization for World War II. This convergence produced a significant expansion in the scope of dietary reform, which came to encompass the entire population, with eating right serving an important social role on the home front. Exploring the nutrition-education component of the World War II home-front food program, I show that lessons in eating right were a means of promoting home-front morale, of delineating wartime ideals of good citizenship, and of reasserting class and gender hierarchies destabilized by wartime social flux.

The second half of the book is framed by postwar shifts in the broader culture of health in the United States, from concerns about contagious diseases to an emphasis on chronic diseases and the behaviors believed to cause or mitigate them, including diet. These changes laid the groundwork for eating habits to move to the center of health discourses in the late twentieth century and early twenty-first, and for eating habits to take on unprecedented levels of social and moral importance for individuals. In the context of growing attention to "lifestyle" in relation to health, a new nutritional paradigm that focused on avoiding or limiting the consumption of particular foods and nutrients gave rise to two very different dietary reform movements: alternative food and the campaign against obesity. In chapter 4 I argue that the mainstream alternative-food movement reproduced the normalizing function of earlier dietary discourses despite its departure from nutritional thinking and embrace of pleasure as a guide for eating right, and that in so doing it actually expanded the purview of dietary reform deeper into the subjectivity of eaters. I also explore the ways in which this movement promoted social ideals that were consistent with ideals of good citizenship that emerged as part of the late-twentieth-century process of neoliberalization. In chapter 5 I focus on the campaign against obesity, which took place against the same social and cultural backdrop. I explore how the ideals of good citizenship produced by the political-economic project of neoliberalism were expressed in this dietary discourse, examining in particular the equating of health with thinness and self-control. In chapter 5 I am especially attentive to how, and why, the social stakes related to obesity have become so consequential, especially for those who are fat.

My arguments are based on my analysis of the discourses of dietary reform—the published and unpublished writings of reformers, as well as the vast and varied materials they produced to bring their messages to the public, from posters to public kitchens. As Patricia Allen explains, "Discourse is what forms and maintains social movement identity. In fact, for some, discourse is primarily what a social movement *is*." Furthermore, Allen writes, "discourse is not only constitutive of social movements; it is also one of the primary tools movements employ to work toward social change."[12] Likewise, discourses are to a large extent what dietary-reform movements *are*—they are the primary tool the reform movements employ toward dietary change—and analysis of these discourses is critical to our ability to understand how our taken-for-granted assumptions about food and health have come to seem so true. The language and practices of dietary reform play an important role in constructing commonsense notions not just about eating right, but also about what it means to be a good person and a good citizen, what health is, and how class operates.

Because I have focused on the discourse of reformers, however, I do not attend to whether or not dietary reform actually affected people's eating habits. I also do not address what the targets of dietary reform thought about it, how they reacted to the dietary advice directed at them, or what "eating right" meant to them. And I risk creating a falsely monolithic sense of what dietary health is and means. I hope that the limits of my analysis incite others to undertake more specific studies of the beliefs and behaviors of communities beyond the dietary-reformers studied here. We need to find and analyze historical evidence of how the assumptions embedded in the discourses I study have been adopted, resisted, and contested by the people who have been the targets of reform, and we need to explore how people who are not reformers have generated and acted on their own "truths" about good food. We also need ethnographic and other kinds of qualitative data that can show us how people of different racial, cultural, and class backgrounds currently understand and use, or refuse, concepts such as "good diet," "good eater," and "eating right" in their everyday lives.

My aim here is to analyze the dynamics of dietary advice, not to give dietary advice, so I don't expect to change anybody's eating habits. But I do intend to change how people think about what it means to eat right. As the voices of the dietary reformers quoted at the beginning of this book suggest, the people who promote dietary advice are hoping to do a lot more than help us each to achieve better health. They see eating habits as a link between individual bodies and the social body, so dietary advice is a way for them to pursue social aims, not just better the health of individuals. While it may often seem like we are each navigating the terrain of dietary choice in purely personal ways that have only to do with our own health and well-being, I hope to have provided a starting point from which to rethink eating right as a social duty, a moral measure, and a form of power worthy of our most critical attention.

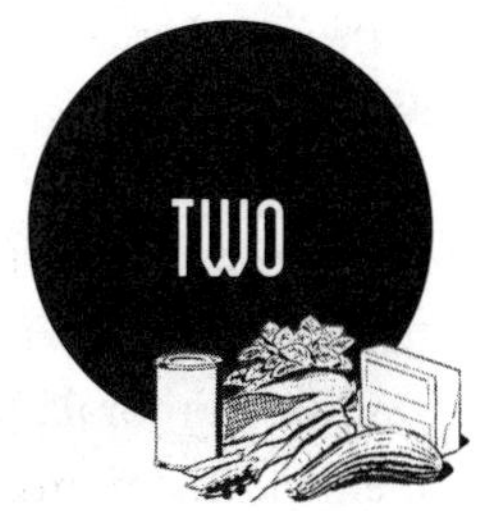

SCIENTIFIC MORALIZATION AND THE BEGINNING OF MODERN DIETARY REFORM

The most recent official dietary advice is MyPlate.[1] Issued by the United States Department of Agriculture (USDA) in 2011, it is designed to make dietary advice simple by showing which foods belong on your plate and in what proportions. The idea is to take the complex facts of nutrition and convey a simple message about diet in a graphic format that connects to how people really think about food. Behind the guide are numbers of accepted truths about the relationship between food, nutrients, and health: that food comprises various nutrients needed by the body, for example, and that each food contains different amounts and kinds of those nutrients; that food delivers calories, which provide energy but are harmful if consumed in larger quantities than the body can use; that certain vitamins are essential to the prevention of diseases and that some can also enhance health. But these basic tenets of nutrition, established and refined over the course of roughly the last 120 years, are only part of what lies behind MyPlate's version of a good diet. MyPlate's simple graphic also expresses a number of beliefs about how people should behave in relation to food, ideas that have been infused with morality since antiquity. Understanding MyPlate or any other dietary advice therefore requires that we look not only at the evolution of nutritional knowledge, but also at the ongoing relationship between nutritional facts and moral precepts.[2]

The science of nutrition provided an empirical accounting of dietary health that was, from its inception, driven by social purpose and suffused with moral intent. Domestic scientists, the first of the modern dietary reformers, leveraged both the empirical and the ethical aspects of nutrition, applying its factual framework to the aims of moral uplift and social amelioration. The failures and idiosyncrasies of these turn of the twentieth century reformers, who championed beef broth and brown bread as a means of moral uplift among the Northeast's urban poor, are well documented. Historians have pointed to the dangerous mistakes in their nutritional calculus, the class-bound conceits of their reform mentalities, and the regressive nature of a gender politics based on domesticity, while acknowledging that the way Americans eat may have been forever transformed by their embrace of science, technology, and industry as essential to modern homemaking.[3] My concern is not whether domestic scientists succeeded or failed in their social mission or how they may have changed American eating habits. Instead it is to investigate the cultural politics of dietary health at the turn of the century so that we might better understand the social role of MyPlate, the Body Mass Index (BMI), or injunctions to "eat local" today. What matters for the present analysis is that domestic science was the first of many twentieth-century dietary reform movements to harness the calculative power of nutritional science for social aims, but its story reveals what the others conceal—the interplay of the moral and the quantitative that is at the core of modern ideals of dietary health. The story of domestic science is critical to understanding the role dietary advice now plays. It is about the formation of a social dynamic of dietary health that has since become part of our common sense, obscured by taken-for-granted notions of what dietary ideals are and do. Domestic scientists took care to articulate the moral valence of eating right, overtly embraced dietary lessons as a way to inculcate social values related to particular ideals of good citizenship, and openly used diet and dietary advice to stabilize the identity of the emerging middle class. I explore each of these facets in turn, illuminating the politics of dietary health that animated the domestic science movement and laying a foundation for seeing subsequent dietary reform movements, and contemporary dietary advice, through a new lens.

Nutrition, Scientific Cookery and the Quantifiable Morality of Eating Right

For people who lived and ate before the ascendance of scientific reasoning, choosing what to eat was mainly a matter of ethical or religious concern. As John Coveney shows, for ancient Greeks practicing ethical comportment in relation to the pleasures of food was instrumental in constructing and displaying an ethical self. Moderation was paramount, but the aim was to enhance, not deny, one's experience of pleasure. Failing to exercise self-mastery and balance between needs and desires was to lose sight of "truth" and "natural reason." For early Christians, strict conduct in relation to food was seen as a duty to God. Pleasure had become a mortal sin and avoiding food pleasure was a way to renounce the flesh and bodily passions. After the Enlightenment, the management of pleasures (related to both food and sex) became the purview of the state, which expressed its rule through medical and scientific discourse. But the concerns that guided writers on diet in the sixteenth and seventeenth centuries—the health of the body, eliminating disease, and the purity of the soul—changed little during the eighteenth and nineteenth centuries. Moral and aesthetic criteria, rather than objective, numerical standards, prevailed.[4]

The language and meaning of eating right were transformed when the emerging science of nutrition produced new ways of measuring the value of food and assessing the wisdom of eating habits. Nutrition produced a quantitative framework and, like other sciences, ultimately staked its claims to authority on the presumed objectivity of the numbers it produced.[5] Its numeric facts made it possible to authoritatively determine a good diet, assess the quality of diets, and compare diets to each other in new ways. But nutrition did not introduce an entirely new conceptualization of the relationship between food and health; it built on existing moral precepts concerning the management of the appetite. The advent of scientific nutrition attached the morality of eating right to a seemingly objective quantitative scaffolding that allowed it to function in new ways. Nutrition provided an objective means of determining good eaters and of numerically assessing and comparing the morality of eaters. I first examine the building blocks of turn-of-the-century nutritional thinking, tracing the social and moral imperatives that drove the knowledge nutrition produced, then follow the trail into the work of domestic scientists, reformers who put nutrition to work for explicitly moral, social purposes.

Wilbur Atwater, "the father of American nutrition," provided three pieces of interlinked information that made possible a new way of thinking about the value of food, the goodness of diets, and the moral character of eaters. In the 1800s, German chemists established that food was comprised of different components that had specific physiological functions (proteins, fats, carbohydrates, and mineral matter).[6] Until the 1880s, balance between these elements was considered the basis for an adequate diet, but the development of the calorie as a means of measuring energy made it possible to more precisely determine a good diet.[7] Atwater, who had trained in Germany and whose federally financed work took place at the first U.S. Experiment Station, in Connecticut, began by investigating and quantifying the chemical components of food. He analyzed 2,600 foods grown and processed in the United States, establishing their chemical composition and organizing the data into tables that showed the amount of water, protein, fat, carbohydrate, "ash" (mineral matter including potassium, sodium, and calcium), and the number of calories, or "fuel value per pound." The tables covered every conceivable cut of meat (from very lean to very fat) and all kinds of other foods, too, from donuts and pies (apple, custard, lemon, mince, and squash) to artichokes (fresh and canned), succotash, lentils, parsnips, peas, apricots, figs, and chocolate.[8] The tables were published by the USDA, and became commonly used among middle-class cooks.[9]

Atwater later put this detailed knowledge of the chemical constituents of thousands of food items into relation to two other pieces of the social and physiological puzzle: the amount of energy that consuming various foods would make available and the cost of each food. He conducted legendary experiments that involved enclosing human subjects in a sealed "calorimeter" and measuring every element that went in as food and water and everything that came out as energy and waste. These efforts revealed what Atwater saw as the "true" value of food—how much energy it could produce as work—and gave the lie to other scales of value. Unpleasant food, it turned out, produced no less energy than did delicious food that was chemically similar. More important, once Atwater had compiled tables that expressed the relationship between energy value and the cost of food, it became clear that the cost of food had no bearing on its nutritional value. The chemicals contained in food had the same effect on, say, a person's ability to ride a stationary bike or perform mathematical computations regardless of how much that food cost.[10] Atwater redefined the value of food based on chemistry and the physiology of human nutrition. But the aim of this computation was not simply to determine what kind of chemicals a given food provided or how much energy would be produced by eating it. It was to better understand the relationship between the nutritional value of food and its cost so that people could be taught to eat well for less. The triangulation of information about the chemical constituents of food, human energy needs, and the cost of foods produced a measure of food value that social reformers embraced precisely because it married the empirical aspects of nutrition to the social and moral aims of economy.[11]

In the late 1880s Atwater published a series of articles in the *Century*, a popular middle-class monthly, in which he discussed the social role of nutritional knowledge. He wanted people to understand that providing their families with good food was not about buying the best, most expensive delicacies, but rather was a matter of understanding the scientific value of food and choosing foods that provided the most energy for work at the least cost. Atwater worried that people of limited means were spending far too much money on food, leaving too little left over for other necessities. He painstakingly explained that the "best food," sold at the highest prices and having the finest flavor, was not necessarily the most economic or the most healthful. He taught readers that using "the protein of oysters to make blood, muscle, and brain will cost him two to three dollars a pound," but the same amount of protein could be had in the form of cod and mackerel for between thirty and eighty cents a pound.[12] Twenty-five cents could buy about 14,000 calories in wheat flour or 12,000 in potatoes.[13] Economizing, not buying expensive food, was the way to improve the diet. Atwater argued that the American view of economy as anathema to "our dignity as free-born" would have to be overcome, and he warned, "Unless we mend our ways the future will bring a loss instead of a gain in material prosperity, and a fearful falling away rather than improvement in our morals."[14] His aim was to "remedy this evil" through "popular understanding of elementary facts regarding food and nutrition, and the acceptance of the doctrine that economy is respectable."[15] The facts of nutrition, combined with the social aim of economy, had produced a quantitative index of dietary morality (see figure 2.1).

Atwater put his knowledge about food to use as a means of moral

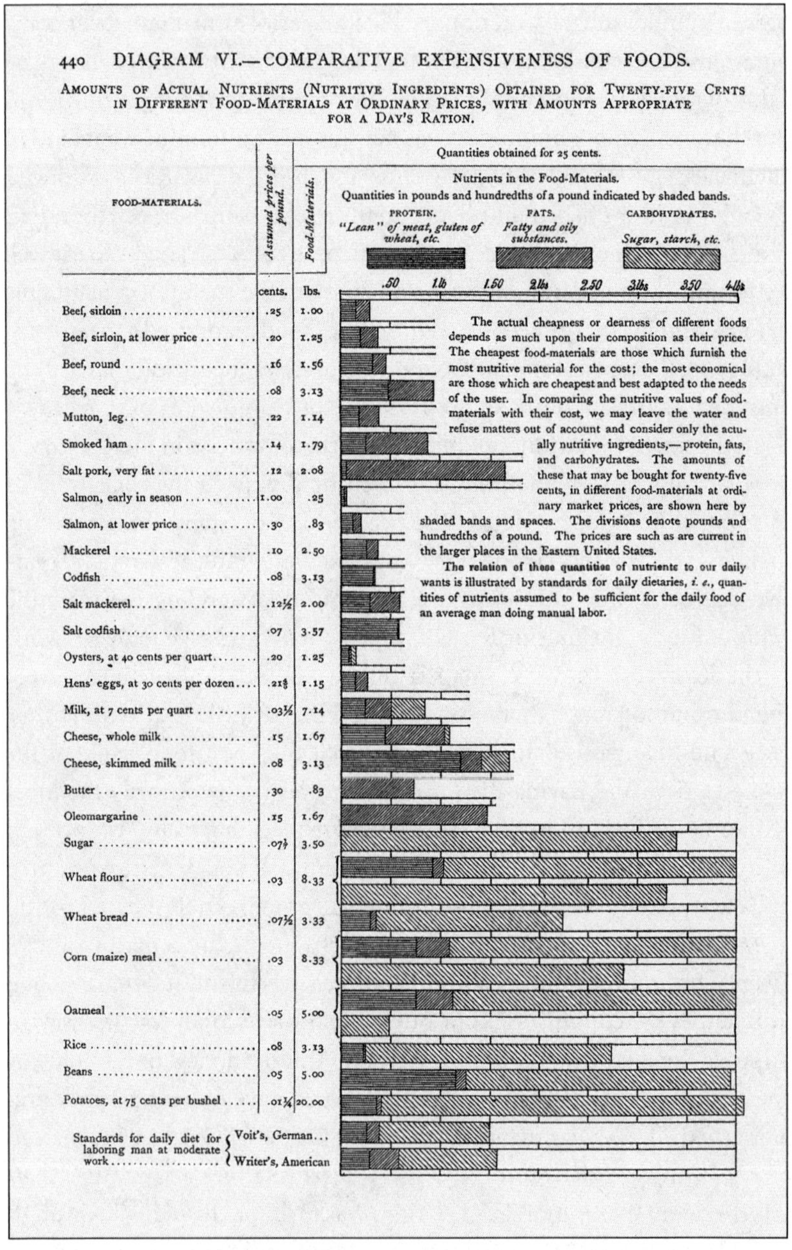

FIGURE 2.1 • W. O. Atwater's "Comparative Expenses of Food," a quantitative index of dietary morality. The subtitle reads: "Amounts of Actual Nutrients (Nutritive Ingredients) Obtained for Twenty-Five Cents in Different Food-Materials at Ordinary Prices, with Amounts Appropriate for a Day's Ration." Courtesy of Cornell University Library, Making of America Digital Collection.

assessment. One of his articles in the *Century*, for example, described a well-meaning coal laborer who did all that he could to provide his family with finest flour and sugar, paid more for the nicest cuts of meat and excellent butter, but therefore had to skimp on other necessities. His family had little left over to pay for new clothes, and they lived in a crowded tenement, sleeping in rooms with no windows, because they "indulged in this extravagance in food."[16] The scientific calculation of food value revealed the moral failings of the coal laborer, who was described by Atwater as "innocently committing an immense economic and hygienic blunder."[17] The blunder was economic, hygienic, and therefore also moral. It was revealed through calculative strategies of nutrition that reflected the values of frugality and self-restraint and that measured dietary health in social and economic terms.

The overt intermingling of nutritional knowledge and moral concern evident in Atwater's work reflected the broader social context of the nineteenth century, in which scientific and religious thought were considered both similar and compatible. As Charles Rosenberg explains, through much of the nineteenth century scientific and religious values were seen as complementary; both offered ideals of selflessness and truth. Moral and scientific progress thus seemed inevitably parallel and complementary. Most nineteenth-century physicians believed, for example, there "could be no conflict between their findings and the truths of morality." Americans typically accepted both realms of thought simultaneously and moved comfortably between them.[18] After the Civil War, science began to garner increasing cultural appeal and prestige. Its processes of counting and calculation came increasingly to be seen, and celebrated, as objective and free of personal values.[19] But a fusion of empiricism and morality was common among turn-of-the-century social movements, which saw female reformers applying the calculative strategies of science and social science to the spectrum of social ills, from intemperance to prostitution. As Rosenberg notes, while "phrased in the measured terms of empirical analysis," these reform movements were "suffused by a vision of transcendent moral benefit."[20]

While some turn-of-the-century reformers launched hygiene and purity campaigns, temperance crusades, playground movements, and tenement reforms, others turned to "the food problem."[21] Enthusiastically embracing nutrition as a simultaneously empirical and moral tool, these women articulated a striking faith in the power of eating right to mitigate the most pressing social concerns of the time. In an 1894 article in the *New England Kitchen*, an organ of the emerging domestic science movement, one reformer wrote, "The proper preparation of food is a vital problem, and the relation of nutriment to personal morality no longer to be ignored. . . . The ministry of diet in the work of character-building is therefore one of the most important studies a woman can undertake."[22] The reformers believed that teaching people to eat right would keep them away from alcohol and labor unions, and improve their character and morals. Drunkenness was seen as a "disease of ill-feeding."[23] Cravings for alcohol were caused by "the constant gnawing of an unsatisfied stomach caused by not having the proper foods properly cooked."[24] Good meals provided in comfortable homes were bound to be more attractive than the street and the saloon, and would mitigate the allure of "rash movements" and protect workingmen from falling prey to "demagogues and partisans."[25] One woman writing about the relationship between diet and "labor problems" explained, "Not only man's physical and mental but his moral well being also depends upon the kind of food he eats." She went on, "By using every possible means to educate the wives and daughters of working men to be more intelligent homemakers, we can do more towards the solution of the labor problem than all the anarchists, the communists, the socialists or even the labor organizations . . . have ever been able to do."[26]

Ellen Richards was among the female reformers who embraced scientific dietary reform as a means of social improvement, and she eventually became their leader and inspiration. An accomplished scientist with a deep appreciation of the moral aspect of eating right, Richards understood the opportunity that the science of food presented for women. Born in 1842, Richards studied chemistry at Vassar, but after graduating in 1870, she was unable to find work in a chemical firm. She applied to Massachusetts Institute of Technology (MIT), then in its infancy, and was admitted as a "special student," becoming the first female to receive a B.S. at that institution (without appearing officially on the books and, therefore, not setting a precedent for coeducation). In 1876 she convinced MIT to establish the Women's Laboratory, where female students worked under her direction until 1883, when they were finally permitted to join the men and Richards was named an instructor of sanitary chemistry, becoming MIT's first female faculty member. As a scientist, Richards was devoted to finding ways of improving domestic life both because she wanted to prove the legitimacy of scientific education for women and because she was convinced that science promised better living. As a reformer, she motivated and directed a groundswell of interest in scientific domesticity, leading the movement that would eventually become home economics. At the time of her death, in 1911, Richards was remembered as the movement's "prophet, its interpreter, its conservator, its inspirer, and to use her own word, its engineer."[27]

Richards's passionate commitment to the application of scientific knowledge toward the aim of creating better homes and cities meant that while she revered the quantifiable norms of a good diet that had been produced by scientific research, she understood them as imparting a clear moral obligation to eat well in the interest of the social order. That she was described as both an engineer and a prophet is entirely fitting, as her commitment to the social application of science was shot through with religious zeal. "We are like wanderers in a dark corridor, dark only because we do not reach up and turn on the light," she wrote, bemoaning the tendency among Americans to refuse to live as well as they might because they had not placed adequate faith in science.[28] Those she inspired also used religious metaphors to describe their project, suggesting that they, too, saw the application of the science of nutrition (and domesticity more broadly) as entirely compatible with religious values. They referred to traveling to give lectures as responding to "a call" or moving to a new city to set up projects as taking up "the work."[29]

The marriage of scientific empiricism to the moral aims of social reform characterized the early work of domestic scientists, who partnered with Atwater on a series of dietary studies and put his nutritional calculations into practice in experimental public kitchens. Working under Atwater's supervision, domestic scientists conducted around 350 studies of the eating habits of American families over a fifteen-year period beginning in 1885. The studies took place in various cities around the country, some were hosted by colleges, and one study, conducted in collaboration with the Tuskegee Normal and Industrial Institute and the Agricultural and Mechanical College of Alabama, focused specifically on "the food of the Negro in Alabama."[30]

In each study the researcher began by accounting for all food materials in a home. Over the course of the next seven days, she measured all food purchased, all kitchen and table waste, and all food remaining at the end. She also observed the content of each meal consumed and, finally, used

Atwater's food composition tables to establish the amount of nutrients being provided. Each study resulted in a table showing the nutrients provided in relation to the costs per person per day. The purpose, Atwater explained, was both to collect information about living conditions and to assess the "pecuniary economy" of the families studied. "Pecuniary economy" referred precisely to the empirical and moral assessment of a family's food choices in terms of how efficiently, or wastefully, they attained energy for work.[31]

Moral assessment was inseparable from the application of the empirical standards of nutritional quantification. The results of each dietary study were passed along to "the woman of the house" in what was called a "frank chat," and also published in USDA bulletins that were read by the growing number of female reformers turning their attention to matters of the diet.[32] The bulletins chronicled the failure of many to economize, and the success of some, whose ability to live well on limited means surprised and impressed the researchers. Moral condemnation was frequently explicit. A mechanic's family living in New York, for example, was described as "shiftless" and "careless" because they were found to be buying "buns at 5 cents a pound when wheat flour was worth 2 cents a pound," and purchasing bananas and oranges, which were "extravagant for people in their circumstances." The researcher who prepared the report noted that the problem was as much one of poor choices as it was one of limited means, writing that "the great trouble here, as in so many poor families of the congested district, lies in unwise expenditures fully as much as in a limited income."[33] The "wisdom" of expenditures was a moral measure that had become quantifiable through the numeric language of nutrition and, therefore, could now be used as a standard for both assessment and comparison.[34]

Domestic scientists embraced nutrition as the guiding principle of every act related to choosing, preparing, serving, and consuming food, but maintained the values of moderation and asceticism that were central to earlier, more overtly ethical approaches to eating right. They saw eating right as a moral practice that began with banishing the sway of tradition, intuition, and preference. They believed American home cooks were too casual, sloppy, and ignorant, and wanted to replace chance with predictability and chaos with a rational, scientific practice consistent with the emerging industrial order. They argued that the kitchen should become a "domestic food laboratory" where the cook practiced "scientific cookery."

As one reformer explained, scientific cookery was considered an extension of the scientific process of digestion, "a long series of processes, essentially digestive outside of the body," which could properly be thought of as "external digestion."[35] While scientific cookery reframed cooking and eating as a scientific process, it was at the same time a moral discourse that moderated pleasure and constrained the possibility of excess in the form of either caloric intake or expense. First and foremost, food was to be conceived of in terms of its function in the body, not its sensual properties or potential to please. Every activity in the "domestic food laboratory" was to be geared toward preparing food to achieve its end: "absorption through the living walls of the alimentary canal to minister to human nutrition."[36] Economy, or the proper correlation between the chemical components of food and the needs of the body, was the guiding principle.

Pleasure was viewed as a threat to the reign of scientific reason in the kitchen, tempting eaters toward both caloric and economic forms of excess. Atwater argued that there was no place for pleasure in the new science of eating right, since taste had no bearing on whether or not food was "healthy and digestible" from a scientific perspective.[37] For domestic scientists, who were more intimately aware of what it really meant to feed people on a daily basis, pleasure was not entirely dispensable, but it had to be moderated through the application of science. As one writer explained, good taste had a role to play, but only because it led to the "greater outpouring of the needed digestive juices, thus furnishing the means for more rapid and complete digestion"—"palatability" was, in essence, an accessory to digestibility.[38] For Richards, the temptations of the appetite were to be reined in by the principles of scientific nutrition. She wrote, "A higher rule of life than the mere gratification of taste, regardless of health and pocket, must prevail" if the "temptation to intemperance in eating was to be resisted," and she described "temperance in the use of foods" as "even more essential than in anything else which tempts man's appetite."[39] She warned that excessive flavor and pleasure were potentially harmful, especially for the young, and argued that infants and children should not be exposed to highly spiced or sweet foods since bad habits could be fixed "by a very little unwise indulgence."[40]

An allegorical tale called "King Palate," published by Mary Hinman Abel in the early 1890s, perfectly illustrates the concerns about managing pleasure that ran through the discourse of scientific cookery. In the story King Palate is a monarch who enjoys himself too much and pays the price until he finally learns to rein in his passions and live within the constraints provided by scientific knowledge. Abel described King Palate as "lawless in his conduct" and doing "just what he pleased," which included enjoying feasts with his subjects. Eventually, his kingdom was overrun by enemies, who went by the names of Indigestion, Dyspepsia, Gout, and "a hundred others." Then Knowledge, a youth of "wondrous promise," arrived, but the king called him a fool and ignored him as long as he could. Eventually, Knowledge grew into a man, developed a following among the people, reined in the passions of the king, and led the land to thrive.[41] In the end, knowledge prevailed over pleasure, just as domestic scientists hoped it would in every American kitchen. The story of King Palate's downfall dramatized the dual function of the dietary advice domestic science promoted, as both a set of empirical rules about what to eat and a set of moral strictures that expressed concerns about moderation and pleasure.

The New England Kitchen, which opened in 1890, put the principles behind this allegorical tale into action. A paragon of scientific cookery in all of its empirical and ethical glory, the New England Kitchen was a public kitchen set up in one of Boston's "poor sections" under the leadership of Richards and Abel.[42] The aim was to provide immigrants and the poor both with pails of food to be taken home and with lessons in eating right that were intended to improve their morals and character. Using Atwater's calculations, Richards and Abel devised a menu of foods to "give the largest possible amount of nourishment for a given amount of money," and they subjected each item to extensive chemical analysis in order to ensure its uniformity and nutritional efficiency.[43] The menu included beef broth, vegetable soup, pea soup, cornmeal mush, boiled hominy, oatmeal mush, pressed beef, beef stew, fish chowder, tomato soup, Indian pudding, rice pudding, and oatmeal cakes. Since most of its patrons were illiterate, the kitchen taught through its food and its example. Its entire operation was open to the view of patrons, who the reformers hoped would learn to appreciate and adopt scientific methods simply through exposure (see figure 2.2). Abel called the kitchen a "silent teacher of cleanliness, intelligent methods, and a uniform and good result in cookery."[44] She explained, "It is good for people to daily pass and sometimes enter a cleanly, pleasant place where . . . they hardly know how, they get hints for more healthful living."[45] In an article on the New England Kitchen in the *Century,* Maria Parloa, a prominent domestic scientist,

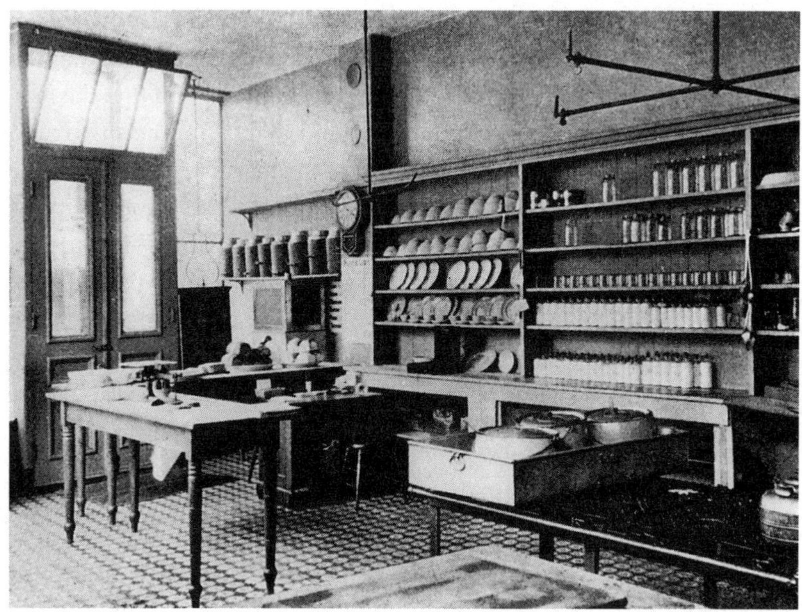

FIGURE 2.2 • A silent teacher: interior of the New England Kitchen. Courtesy of the MIT Museum.

celebrated its intertwined material and ethical aims, writing that when people with poor diets "are educated up to the point where they choose soups, well-cooked cereals, and good milk, there will be a great gain in their physical and moral condition."[46]

After an initial period of excitement, in the mid-1890s the reformers who had invested so much in the conceptualization and materialization of the public kitchens noticed that the population they aimed to reach had little appetite for the scientific morality they were serving. Philanthropic support waned, kitchens either closed or abandoned their original missions, and domestic scientists began to come to terms with the fact that they would have to give up their attempts to reform the poor and invest their attention elsewhere.[47] In trying to understand why their project failed, Abel and the others noted that their patrons were simply unwilling to cede their own measures of good food to scientific standards.

Richards noticed that the intended patrons rejected the New England Kitchen not simply because they did not like the food it offered, but also because they were not willing to accept the definition of eating right that it embodied and sought to transmit. She wrote that the "death knell" of the public kitchens was sounded "by the woman who said 'I don't want to eat what's good for me; I'd ruther eat what I'd ruther,'" and that the man who pointed to a baked Indian pudding and said, "'You needn't try to make a Yankee of me by making me eat that' . . . may have helped ring the knell."[48] The kitchen offered a menu of food that was "good" by the measure of scientific nutrition but not necessarily so by the measures of taste, tradition, and cultural status that were meaningful to the men and women, many of them immigrants, who it sought to serve.[49] Levenstein has detailed the "manifest failings" of the reformers: they failed to appreciate that working-class families considered better food (especially more beefsteak) the just reward of their hard work; they suffered from "bland palates and underdeveloped appreciations of the joy of eating"; and they studiously ignored the tastes of their immigrant customers.[50] But the reformers sought to impose a bland New England diet not merely out of insensitivity and ignorance. Rather, they were redefining the meaning of eating right through the lens of science and learning to quantify the morality of eating right.

The failure of the public kitchens did not stop the momentum of domestic science; it merely launched the movement into its next, more successful phase. And despite its failure to achieve its stated intent—to improve the diets and character of immigrants and the poor—the early work of the domestic science movement represented an important transition in the culture of dietary health. The dietary studies and the public kitchens applied ideals that married morality and scientific nutrition, making them the first modern dietary-reform projects. The ideals of a good diet that provided the most nutrition at the least possible cost and a cooking practice that scientifically reduced pleasure to its chemical role in digestion introduced a new meaning of eating right that was infused with moral asceticism but spoke in the increasingly authoritative, numeric language of science, making a good diet for the first time a seemingly objective, quantifiable moral measure.

"Natural Law" and the Making of Good Citizens

While we tend to think about choosing a good diet as a matter of individual bodily health, because of the moral content of dietary ideals eating right is also a process of self-assessment, self-improvement, and self-making that takes place in relation to particular social values, norms, and ideals.[51] As efforts to improve the eating habits and the character of the Northeast's urban poor lost momentum in the mid-1890s, Ellen Richards began to connect the empiricism of nutrition and scientific cookery to the particular social ideals of Progressivism, and to articulate the moral dimension of nutrition in relation to emerging ideals of good citizenship. Concerns about intemperance gave way to pronouncements about race improvement and the importance of learning to sacrifice individual liberty for the sake of "true democracy." In the first decade of the twentieth century Richards and her allies built a movement, known as home economics, that taught people to eat right and, in the process, instilled emerging norms of good citizenship. Home economics leveraged the ethical aspects of dietary advice to help acclimate the public to massive changes in social conditions and the structure and function of the federal government; it was as much about training citizens for the Progressive Era as it was about teaching the science of domesticity.

Richards's ideas about the social role that domestic science should play were initially out of sync with the aims of many of her colleagues, who were motivated by an entirely different and more mundane concern—the servant shortage caused by the proliferation of jobs in the growing industrial sector. They were focused on teaching cooking and sewing to inexperienced girls and on training middle-class women to better manage their servants or make do with less help. Richards redirected the movement by assembling people who shared her motives, with the hope that they might eventually form a new organization to replace the National Household Economics Association (NHEA), which focused on securing skilled labor for middle-class homes.[52] In 1899 she organized a meeting of a small group of like-minded reformers in Lake Placid, New York. The eleven attendees chose "home economics" as a name for their work and discussed training teachers, developing high-school curricula, and the need for showing colleges and universities the importance of the new field.[53] The conference accomplished what Richards had hoped it would, setting into motion a reorientation of the domestic-science community around addressing social problems through interventions into the educational system. Home-economics reformers continued to meet annually in Lake Placid for the next ten years. Attendees, who eventually numbered close to seven hundred, included instructors and supervisors of programs in domestic science from kindergarten to college, magazine editors, women running dietary programs in sanatoriums and hospitals, Canadian and English leaders in the field, and a few men with relevant expertise such as, on occasion, Wilbur Atwater.[54] By 1903 the NHEA had collapsed, and six years later the American Home Economics Association was formed, with Richards as its first president. By 1914 home-economics courses were offered in 250 colleges and universities, with 28 four-year programs leading to a bachelor's degree, 20 masters programs, and one doctoral program in household administration.[55]

Despite its reputation as a short-sighted effort to teach cooking and cleaning, home economics in its foundational period was a reform movement with social aims that were shaped in part by widespread concerns about "the future of the race."[56] As the public kitchens failed, Richards shifted focus away from working with the urban poor and toward dietary reform among the middle class in the name of race betterment. In 1899, as she neared the culmination of this gradual transition, she explained: "I believe that the greatest need of intelligent persons today is a right attitude of mind towards the development of the highest powers of the human race. I believe that the well-to-do classes are being eliminated by their diet, to the detriment of social progress, and *they* and *not* the poor are the most in need of missionary work."[57] Like many of her contemporaries, Richards feared that modern life was destroying the vigor and reproductive vitality of the Anglo-Saxon middle class. Darwinism had created a consciousness of species, an awareness of well-being at the level of race, and a new obligation to be healthy for the sake of the race. An ambiguous term, *race* could refer to the human race, to a nation or population, or to a distinct social unit, much like the term *class*. While in the context of Progressive Era health reform *race* ostensibly applied to the human race in general, it was understood by most to have a special reference to Anglo-Saxons.[58] The concept of health as a duty to the race at the turn of the century implied, therefore, that the Anglo-Saxon portion of the population should regenerate itself and then "rescue the less blessed (and potentially race destroying) portions of humankind."[59] The eugenics movement generated and capitalized on this concern, channeling widespread social anxiety into a program for improving the future of the race. Eventually, eugenics consolidated around sexual selection as the most important means of race betterment, advocating both positive (encouraging better breeding) and negative (eliminating the unfit) methods of improving heredity. But prior to World War I, efforts to improve the environments in which people lived also played an important role. Many saw environmental reform as an important corollary to hereditary reform.[60]

For Richards, dietary reform was a way to improve individuals in the present, rather than wait for the effects of eugenic reform on future generations. Richards began to develop her thinking on the relationship of diet to race betterment in the early 1890s and refined her analysis throughout the next two decades, finally publishing a book on the concept in 1910. In 1901 Richards wrote, "In the interest of the race, of its mental as well as physical development, there is no subject which should occupy the attention of educators comparable with that of food and its influence on human progress."[61] In 1904 she explained to her colleagues at the Lake Placid Conference that the word *eugenics* had been coined by Francis Galton to express a better race, and she suggested the term *euthenics* to describe better living. "Euthenics," she argued, should be used instead of "home economics" as a name for the work that was being done in higher education.[62] At the 1906 Lake Placid Conference, Richards explained that euthenics was "the science of better living conditions in order that the human race may enter into its heritage of fuller organic life, instead of sinking below the beasts of the field."[63] Her thinking on the topic culminated with the publication, shortly before her death, of *Euthenics: The Science of a Controllable Environment*, in which she described euthenics as focusing on the "better raised" instead of the "better born."[64] "Euthenics precedes eugenics," she wrote, "developing better men now, and thus inevitably creating a better race of men in the future. Euthenics is the term proposed for the preliminary science on which eugenics must be based."[65] Euthenics was hygiene not for future generations but for "the present generation," and while eugenics was awaiting "careful investigation," euthenics presented "immediate opportunity."[66] Dietary reform was resolutely central to this vision of race progress. "The food problem is fundamental to the welfare of the race," Richards wrote in *Euthenics*. "Society, to protect itself, must take cognizance of the question of food and nutrition."[67]

Richards's euthenics, with its passionate commitment to social betterment through changes to living conditions, was entirely consistent with the aims and tactics of the Progressive movement.[68] In fact, the dietary ideals articulated within the framework of home economics conveyed core ideals of Progressivism, using the language of eating right to help reframe notions of freedom and democracy and to prepare Americans for a new iteration of what it meant to be a good citizen. Richards argued that the public schools, founded for "the production of efficient citizens," were failing to fulfill their mandate because they had not adapted to the changing needs of American society. She explained that while lessons in the three Rs—reading, 'riting, and 'rithmetic—may have once been sufficient, there was now a need for "a fourth R in addition to the time honored three . . . *Right Living*."[69] She advocated lessons in Right Living, or "right ideals of life and its meaning," that would train good citizens by giving "every child the means of making himself an efficient human being."[70]

These lessons in Right Living were to be delivered through a rigorous scientific education that emphasized, above all, the importance of understanding and submitting to the laws of nature. For Richards and her colleagues, the concept of natural law, or the laws of nature, referred to principles that governed the natural world.[71] Especially in the high-school curriculum, learning the laws of nature was emphasized over learning practical lessons. Students in a high-school home-economics course might spend ten weeks on physics, twenty on chemistry, and a mere three to eight weeks applying the science in planning and cooking meals.[72] Though usually remembered as being as fluffy as the cakes they aspired to perfect, early home-economics courses delivered (mostly to young girls) a serious education in natural law and, concurrently, in the social values of Progressivism.[73]

Richards, who described home economics as "nothing less than an effort to save our social fabric from what seems inevitable disintegration," had a profound appreciation for the kind of unity and order that the laws of nature could impose on the chaos of contemporary life.[74] For Richards and her colleagues the universal laws of nature seemed to offer a way to renew the social cohesion that industrialization and urbanization had so badly frayed.[75] The question of what held the society together concerned many Americans at the turn of the century, as they experienced a disorienting transition from the agricultural rhythms and familiar relationships of small-town life to the dizzying industrial pace and complex social networks of the urban context. Some turned to natural law to explain and impose cohesion.[76] The notion that there existed a set of irrefutable laws whose proof could be seen throughout the natural world, but particularly in the body, appealed to members of the middle class for whom the cultural and political changes of the nineteenth century were overwhelming.[77] Richards and her colleagues, for example, noted that projects such as the New England Kitchen could not succeed because of the unmanageable heterogeneity of the urban population. The diverse tastes and "national preferences" of those dwelling within Northeastern cities simply could not be pleased by a single menu. The laws of nature, however, offered to contain and order the chaos of diverse tastes, preferences, and habits. As Mary Hinman Abel explained not long after the failure of the kitchens, "To the unlearned man every food stands by itself and is only to be judged by its taste; but science has reduced the seeming complexity to order."[78] An unwavering set of truths that emanated from nature and was ordained by the authority of science helped to limit the available interpretations of a "good diet." Science offered a set of beautifully irrefutable truths that, many hoped, would reduce dissent and structure the increasingly complex society.

Through the teaching of natural law, home-economics courses conveyed lessons in good citizenship similar to those being taught in civics courses. The role of the national government had historically been to collect taxes and appropriate funds, but by the end of the nineteenth century Progressive reformers were beginning to envision and create a professionally staffed government broadly involved in managing the operation of society.[79] In response, a new civics curriculum treated the notion of individual liberty as a myth that needed to be replaced by acceptance of government's role in curtailing individual freedom for the sake of society.[80] For home economics, the laws of nature provided irrefutable proof that man was not intended for unregulated freedom and a means of instilling the habit of willing compliance with the increasingly interventionist laws of the growing state. Reflecting changes in notions of citizenship related to the legal separation of citizenship from suffrage, civics education was no longer about voting and political rights, focusing instead on moral education, teaching a sense of dependence and deference to experts, and developing desirable habits and behaviors (including health habits).[81] Home economics also taught exactly these things, using the notion of natural law as a means of instilling an ethos of obedience and deference to experts while training pupils in Right Living, the habits of daily life that would best express self-control and morality.

Like civics courses, home-economics courses paved the way for the state-building endeavors of the Progressive Era, teaching reliance on government and limiting the notion of individualism to fit within the growing need for an active state and the expansion of government regulation and welfare programs. Richards adamantly supported the growing role of the federal government, explaining, "Conditions of motion, of rapid intermingling of distant populations" demanded "national control" through "prompt and thorough action which well-equipped Federal forces alone possess."[82] In 1900, at the second Lake Placid Conference, Richards described home economics as a means of preparing students for a form of citizenship that emphasized responsibility to the needs of the larger social group and required obedience to natural laws and by extension to the laws of the state. She talked about the importance of developing a child's responsibility toward his environment, of teaching him about his relationship to "public health and public morals," and of helping him to understand "the laws that govern the moral and physical health of the individual, and of his obligation to keep these laws."[83] In *Euthenics* she wrote an eloquent defense of the ideals of Progressivism that animated home economics: "The individual may be wise to his own needs, but powerless by himself to secure the satisfaction of them. Certain concessions to others' needs are always made in family life. The community is only a larger family group."[84] She went on to explain that with new regulations helping to manage the life of the community, it was no longer reasonable to expect the same kind of freedom; by coming into the community, the individual "forfeited his right to unrestrained individuality."[85]

Richards had long believed that the American ethos of individualism needed to be revised to make way for new political realities and that the teaching of natural law, while potentially unwelcome, offered a way of doing so. In *The Cost of Food* (1901), she bemoaned the difficulty of teaching Right Living, "especially in the face of the intense individualization so widely taught—namely that each person is a law unto himself."[86] She expressed concern that her efforts to teach respect for natural law were so often met with "scoffing" and "a demand for freedom and unrestrained choice as a mark of American Liberty."[87] Expressing her frustration, she continued, "Men have yet to learn that 'independence cannot with safety be made to apply to their relations with nature.'"[88] Richards argued passionately for a more limited interpretation of freedom, and saw lessons in Right Living as an obvious means of instilling them into the daily lives of Americans. She explained that most Americans had a mistaken notion of liberty as meaning "each person is a law unto himself"; on the contrary, she argued, true freedom came not from "unrestrained choice" but from living knowledgeably within the constraints provided by "the fixed principles which govern all living organisms."[89] Obedience to natural law was especially important when it came to food, and Richards saw home economics as an opportunity to teach people how to eat not just for themselves, but for the good of the whole. At the fourth Lake Placid Conference, she explained, "Each man likes to be law unto himself in the first flush of freedom. He thinks that is democracy. But the student finds that true democracy is sacrifice for the sake of many. In food, not what *we like* but what is good for the many should be the standard."[90]

That lessons in eating right were also lessons in natural law, which were truly lessons in good Progressive Era citizenship, was beautifully illustrated by a report presented by the Committee on Home Economics in the Elementary and Secondary Schools at the third Lake Placid Conference, in 1901. The committee expressed concern that their students thought freedom meant the liberty to do whatever they wanted, and complained that this led to "a certain lawlessness," "lack of personal responsibility," and "deplorably bad manners."[91] The report went on to explain how a lesson in bread baking could remedy these problems by teaching students about the absolute limits on freedom that natural law imposed. Sure, the girls were free individuals, but if they simply did as they pleased—"refuse to pour boiling water on the yeast, forget the salt, refuse to make their muscles work effectively, let the dough stand a length of time convenient to themselves, and fail to manage the oven dampers"—they would learn the consequences of disobeying the laws of nature. They would find that "Nature has gone quietly on her way, and returns to them their just due; their own careless, irresponsible selves expressed in a soggy, dark, sour, ill shaped loaf of bread." Such a lesson, the committee explained, would result in much more than better bread. They described the lesson as one that put "in concrete terms the whole matter of the limitation of the individual by his environment," arguing that "through a series of such experiences there comes an understanding of what law means, and self-control, and obedience, and freedom."[92]

Eating Right and the Making of the Middle Class

In a space large enough to seat just thirty people at a time, ten thousand attendees of the 1893 World's Columbian Exhibition in Chicago were served a scientifically calibrated lunch in an exact replica of the New England Kitchen (see figures 2.3 and 2.4). The Rumford Kitchen served brown bread, pea soup, beef broth, "escalloped fish," rolls, gingerbread, and

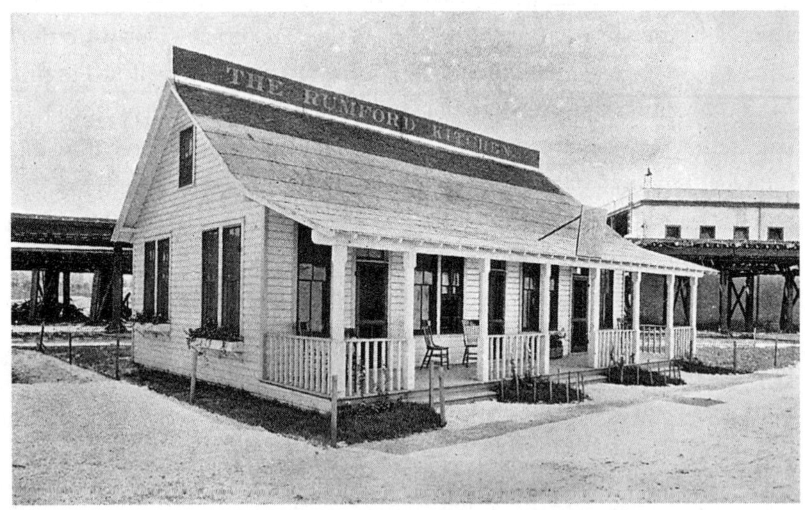

FIGURE 2.3 • The Rumford Kitchen at the World's Columbian Exhibition. Courtesy of MIT Libraries, Institute Archives and Special Collections, Cambridge, Massachusetts, Report of Massachusetts Board of World's Fair Managers, World's Columbian Exposition, Chicago, 1893.

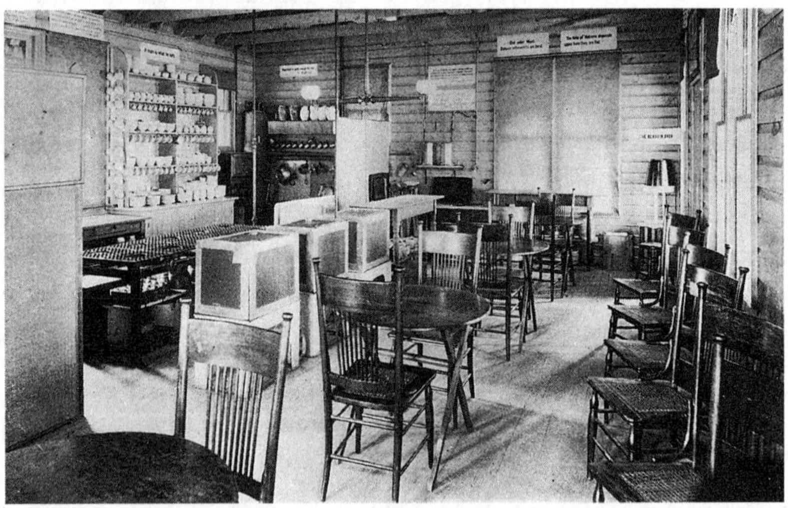

FIGURE 2.4 • Interior of the Rumford Kitchen, with mottos visible on the walls. Courtesy of MIT Libraries, Institute Archives and Special Collections, Cambridge, Massachusetts, Report of Massachusetts Board of World's Fair Managers, World's Columbian Exposition, Chicago, 1893.

baked apples, but it was decidedly not a restaurant.[93] Like the New England Kitchen, the operation was not about feeding people so much as it was about teaching them to eat right; it was an "absolutely scientific and educational" enterprise dedicated to the "application of science to the preparation of food." But while the New England Kitchen had attempted to reform the urban poor, the aim of the Rumford Kitchen was to "arouse the intelligent, thinking citizen to the need and possibility of improving in these directions."[94] The reproduction of the New England Kitchen in this new context was meant to demonstrate the basics of scientific nutrition and scientific cookery to a new audience, but it served another purpose as well: to highlight and dramatize the distinction between the "incorrigible poor" and the eager, amenable "intelligent classes." The middle-class audience at the fair turned out to be much easier to teach, in part because they were literate—there were menu cards on each table showing the relationship between daily nutritional requirements and the composition of each dish being served, blocks demonstrating the composition of the human body, a reference library on food and hygiene, and inspirational quotations lining the walls.[95] But the fairgoers also proved themselves to be much more amenable to scientific eating than were urban slum dwellers. Drawing out this distinction gave the reformers an opportunity to define and distinguish the middle-class patrons of the Rumford Kitchen as good eaters in contrast to the immigrants and urban poor whose stubbornness has caused the New England Kitchen to fail.

Just as the introduction of nutritional quantification made eating habits available as a mode of comparison between individuals, so, too, did it provide a means for creating, identifying, and comparing social classes on the basis of how well they managed to attain the goal and social ideal of dietary health. The middle class emerged as a social identity and style of living in the nineteenth century, as certain "daily routines and social networks" distinguished the lives of some people from those of others above and below them in the social hierarchy.[96] But even as the term *middle class* was achieving a relatively stable and widely understood meaning toward the end of the nineteenth century, the concept, according to one historian, "crumbled at the touch."[97] Changes in the structure and scale of capitalism were undermining class distinctions based on the difference between manual and nonmanual labor, blurring the boundary between middle-class "brain workers" and the hard-working laboring class. The expansion of permanently low-paying nonmanual jobs and a severe economic depression between 1873 and 1896 meant that many who might have expected to attain middle-class status were unable to do so.[98] The middle class was at once expanding in size and searching for ways to know and distinguish itself that transcended increasingly unreliable economic and occupational markers.

The pursuit of health became a means for the professionalizing middle class of the late nineteenth and early twentieth centuries to know and identify itself and to stake claims to responsibility and authority. Health became a key marker of middle-class morality and identity, but its utility as such derived in large part from the way it could distinguish members of the responsible middle class from those beneath them in the social hierarchy who failed to achieve the goal of health. Robert Crawford explains that the identity of the "healthy self derived from two interrelated oppositions: "(1) a biologically healthy self that is conceived in opposition to disease and death; and (2) a metaphorically healthy self by way of which conventional beliefs about the self are imagined as opposed to the qualities of 'unhealthy' persons *already* positioned as subordinate, outside, and stigmatized."[99] The "unhealthy other," positioned as outside, stigmatized and dangerous, was a common figure in the discourse of health reform at the turn of the century. Tuberculosis crusades, for example, appealed to stereotypes of the other as "dirty and dangerous" despite public rhetoric emphasizing the democratic intent of health education. "Not surprisingly," writes Nancy Tomes, "the 'careless' or 'unteachable' consumptive was usually poor, uneducated, and foreign-born or nonwhite."[100]

Domestic scientists began to both assert and leverage the significance of the distinction between the healthy middle class and the unhealthy other as they celebrated the "resounding success" of the Rumford Kitchen. In addition to bringing scientific meals to thousands of fairgoers, the Rumford Kitchen presented a moment in which failure of the poor to live by the new knowledge of nutrition was set into stark contrast with the apparently avid interest of the "intelligent classes" in eating right. Among the twenty printed leaflets distributed at the kitchen and later published as *The Rumford Kitchen Leaflets*, there were two pieces in which Mary Hinman Abel reflected on the difficulties the reformers faced trying to change the diets of "working men" and contrasted this to the ease with which the middle-class audience was reached.[101] "The Story of the New England Kitchen" and "Public Kitchens in Relation to the Working Man and the Housewife" detailed the stubbornness and lack of interest among the poor that had in

Abel's opinion led to the demise of the public kitchens. Abel portrayed the poor as unreachable, "incorrigible," and too diverse to be pleased by a single menu. She wrote that the problems of the public kitchens primarily arose from a single cause: "The extreme slowness with which the mass of people change their habits with regard to food." She went on to very directly point out the contrast between the stubborn class and the more flexible class: "The cosmopolitan traveler and the fashionable diner-out will taste of a new dish with readiness, while the factory worker or the average school girl cannot be brought to try it." The success of the Rumford Kitchen was taken as further proof that the middle class was unlike the "large class" of people who refused to eat what was good for them and who opted instead to eat what they liked.[102] Recognizing the middle class as open to reform in contrast to the stubborn "unhealthy other," domestic scientists provided advice about how to eat right that helped to further define middle-class identity and delineate its boundaries.

Maintaining the fuzzy boundaries of the new middle class entailed taking into account all of the factors that worked together to define its common experience and outlook. The dietary ideals that domestic scientists promoted did exactly this by defining a good diet as eating habits that were accurately calibrated to the income, occupation, experience, lifestyle, and habituated preference of the eater.[103] The notion that a good diet was different for people with different incomes was the fundamental premise of early nutrition and the reform movement that promoted its principles. It was precisely the inappropriate expenditure on food relative to income that Atwater wanted to remedy through his research, which revealed that there was no reason to spend a meager income on expensive sources of energy when less-expensive sources were available. Atwater's research established the fact that the cost of food, as Richards explained, "is no measure of its nutritive value."[104] One of the Rumford Kitchen leaflets celebrated this odd but wonderful fact: "How strange it seems the fact, when we first learn it, that a Roman feast and a Lenten feast, a Delmonico dinner and the lunch of a wayside beggar, all contain the same few simple elements of nutrition! . . . So this is nature's democracy, food is food, for a' the wit of cooks!"[105] "Nature's democracy" made it both irrational and immoral to choose expensive cuts of meat and other delicacies if means were limited, but doing so was perfectly appropriate, in fact expected, when money was available.

Domestic scientists conveyed the importance of dietary differentiation by income to the American public. They provided books, leaflets, lectures and school curricula that reiterated Atwater's principles of nutritional efficiency and taught women how to provide good diets at various costs per day and for various income levels. For example, Richards's book *The Cost of Food: A Study in Dietaries* delineated proper diets for people at several different income levels. For those subsisting on fifteen cents per person per day Richards recommended an evening meal consisting of milk, homemade bread, butter, and stewed pears, while for those spending one dollar a day tomato soup, halibut, filet of beef with piquant sauce, potatoes, beets, sweetbreads, and lady fingers were among the items on the menu (see figures 2.5 and 2.6).[106]

Anxiety lurked at the heart of this eminently practical advice, which reflected not only Atwater's aim of keeping the working classes happy on limited incomes in order to avoid social unrest, but also the social concerns of reformers who recognized the fluidity and instability of class markers. A series of articles published in the mid-1890s in the movement's magazine, *New England Kitchen*, expressed concerns about "dishonesty in caste" and urged readers to dress, eat, entertain, furnish their homes, and approach housekeeping with "honesty." The articles repeatedly stressed that people should not attempt to deceive others by adopting the food, clothing, or home décor of another class. In her first article the author Ethel Davis explained that "correct analysis of social position is absolutely necessary to the perfect furnishing of a home . . . No surroundings, no occupation, no circumstances of environment can change the proper classification of a human being in the social world."[107] The notion of honesty in class meant that people should eat in appropriate relation to their actual means, and that a wife should not offer food to guests that might present a deceptive picture of her "husband's position." Give them "sweet-breads and quail if that is what you can afford to supply for your household and them," urged the author, "bread and molasses if that is your alternative."[108]

Teaching people to choose meals and menus that reflected their income was but one aspect of how domestic scientists leveraged the discourse of dietary health as a means of identity making and boundary marking for the middle class. Part of the problem facing the middle class was that income was no longer a reliable means of distinguishing the middle class. The manual-nonmanual divide initially provided the foun-

DIETARIES COSTING TEN TO FIFTEEN CENTS 109

TABLE X

Dietary No. 1

FOR AVERAGE FAMILY OF SIX, 15 CENTS PER PERSON PER DAY

	Lbs.	Oz.	Gms.	Cost.	Grams.			Cal.
					Prot.	Fat.	Carb.	
Breakfast.								
Baking-powder biscuit				$0.10	72.2	39	447	2491
Ham (lean)	1		453	.15	81.5	85		1123
Butter		1⅓		.025	.2	36		333
Potatoes	2			.02	16	.8	138	650
Milk for coffee			160	.01	6	7	8	122
Sugar for coffee			60	.007			60	246
				0.312	175.94	168	653	4965
Dinner.								
Beef-shank stew	3		1360	0.24	185	53		1251
Potatoes	1			.01	8	.4	69	325
Turnips	1			.02	4.5	.5	28	138
Thickening				.015	7.5	24.7	53	477
Suet pudding:								
Beef-suet	½			.03		220		2040
1 qt. flour				.028	66	6	428	2056
1 cup molasses				.02			113	463
Soda, sweet sauce				.01		10	50	298
				0.373	271	314.6	741	7048
Supper.								
Milk, 1 pint				0.03	15	18	22.7	325
Bread (home-made) and butter				.10	61	126.5	319	2734
Stewed pears				.045	4	5	216	962
				0.175	80	149.5	557.7	4021
Totals:								
Breakfast				.312	176	168	653	4965
Dinner				.373	271	314.6	741	7048
Supper				0.175	80	149.5	557.7	4021
				0.86	537	632.1	1951.7	16034
Tea, coffee, etc.				.04				
				0.90				
Per person				.15	89.5	105.3	325.3	2672

453.6 grms = 1 lb.
1 grm. proteid and carbohydrates = 4.1 calories.
1 grm. fat = 9.3 calories.

FIGURE 2.5 • "Dietary No. 1: For Average Family of Six, 15 Cents per Person per Day." Ellen Richards, *The Cost of Food: A Study of Dietaries* (New York: J. Wiley and Sons, 1901).

142 THE COST OF FOOD

TABLE XXIV

DIETARY NO. 5

$1.00 PER PERSON PER DAY

	Lbs.	Oz.	Gms.	Cost.	Grams.			Cal.
					Prot.	Fat.	Carb.	
Breakfast.								
Strawberries	3	.....	.....	$0.40	12	8	83	465
Sugar	.....	5.6	159	.018	.....	.....	159	652
Cream of wheat	.....	.....	127	.02	13	2.5	96.6	472
Cream	.....	.....	230	.15	6	61	6.5	618
Eggs (9)	.....	18	505	.24	60	47	.....	836
French rolls (1 dozen)	1	.....	453	.12	44	24	260	1465
Butter	.....	3	84	.12	8	72	.....	700
Coffee	.....	1	28.3	.025				
Sugar	.....	2	60	.007	.....	.....	60	246
Thick cream	.....	.....	115	.075	3	30.5	3.3	309
				1.175	146	245	668.4	5763
Luncheon.								
Chicken (broiled)	4	.....	.....	1.00	268	20	.....	1300
Butter, 2 tbs.*	.....	.....	28	.015	.....	24	.....	224
Potato chips.	0.5	.....	.....	.05	17	80	115	1290
Cold asparagus (salad)	2	.....	.....	.30	16	1.8	29.9	210
French dressing (½ cup of oil)	.....	.....	.....	.08	.....	120.2	.....	1118
Bread	.....	.....	200	.02	19	3	108	544
Tea	.....	½	.....	.03	.....	.....	.....	.....
Sugar	.....	2	.....	.007	.....	.....	60	246
Cherries	1	.....	453	.10	.....	.....	66	260
Gingerbread (thin)	.....	.....	250	.04	16	32	124	852
				1.642	336	281	503	6044
Dinner.								
Tomato soup	2	.....	.....	.10	62.2	10	50.8	370
Halibut, creamed	.....	.....	.....	.278	76.4	43	23.3	765
Bread for the whole dinner	.....	.....	200	.02	19	3	108	544
Filet of beef, piquant sauce	3	.....	.....	1.00	234	252	.....	3300
Potatoes	1	.....	.....	.02	.8	.4	68	315
New beets	0.5	.....	.....	.10	4.8	.4	17.4	170
Sweetbread and cucumber salad (No. 30), mayonnaise dressing	.....	.....	.....	.73	79	194	17.5	2030
Saltines	.....	1	28	.025	2.9	.....	24	110
Café parfait (home-made)	.....	.....	.....	.475	12	122	214	1956
Lady-fingers	.....	.....	4	.05	7	11	80	457
Coffee	.....	1	.....	.025				
Sugar	.....	2	.....	.007	.....	.....	60	246
Olives, relishes, garnishes, etc	.....	.....	.....	.35				
Total	.....	.....	.....	3.18	498	635.8	663.0	10263
				6.00	980	1161.8	1834.4	22070
Per person	.....	.....	.....	1.00	163	193.6	305.7	3678
Less 15 per cent of waste oil, fat, and sugar—on plates, in coffee, etc	.....	.....	.....	.....	24	29	46	552
					139	164	259	3126

* tbs. = tablespoonful.

FIGURE 2.6 • "Dietary No. 5: $1.00 per Person per Day." Ellen Richards, *The Cost of Food: A Study of Dietaries* (New York: J. Wiley and Sons, 1901).

dation for the economic distinction between the middle class of brain workers and the working class of laborers. But nonmanual employment no longer guaranteed an income consistent with middle-class lifestyle. In the context of this boundary confusion, domestic scientists promoted dietary advice that reaffirmed the distinction between brain workers and muscle workers. Atwater's work with the "calorimeter" laid the foundation for dietary ideals that differentiated between the needs of people doing different kinds of work. The calorimeter allowed Atwater to measure all the energy that entered in the form of food, drink, and oxygen and all the energy that exited in the form of carbonic acid, water, and "the products of elimination." Atwater also used the calorimeter to investigate the amount of food that was required to sustain the body weight of a subject as he engaged in different kinds of activity. He had subjects perform "severe mental labor" (computing the results of previous experiments and studying a German treatise on physics) and "severe muscular work" (raising and lowering weights for eight hours, three days in a row) in the calorimeter.[109] Atwater explained that he hoped his findings would lead to a better understanding of the "kinds and amounts [of food] which are appropriate for people of different classes and under different circumstances."[110] Building on these findings, domestic scientists stressed that good diets needed to reflect not only income but also occupation. As one reformer explained in an 1896 lecture, "The food for the father of the family must be adapted to his employment. The man whose labor is out of doors and muscular rather than mental, will require the larger bulk of food and it may be composed of the kind least easy of digestion. The indoor laborer needs a very different diet."[111]

But the advice went beyond the empirical need for more calories among those doing physically strenuous work, taking into account the taste and lifestyle aspects of class as well. Richards, for example, suggested that brain-workers such as professors, students, doctors, and teachers should be given a "liberal, varied, well-cooked, and, especially, well-flavored" diet. Their food should be "delicately served with all the attractiveness of napery and china," and neatness and suitability of temperature should be carefully attended to. Manual workers such as housekeepers, janitors, nurses, cooks, and maids, on the other hand, should be given hearty food in few courses, and they should never be fed soups or salads. "What we would call heavy food will not harm these vigorous hard workers," wrote Richards.[112] She also made it clear, however, that in cases where the two aims conflicted, maintaining class distinctions was more important than maintaining the manual-mental distinction. She argued, for example, that even when middle- and upper-class people engaged in physical activity, they needed to eat differently from working people who engaged in physical activity; active youth needed more energy than did sedentary brain workers, but that did not mean that the Harvard boat crew should eat the same foods as youths in a logging camp or soldiers in the field. Excessive physical activity required a lot of food energy but, Richards explained, the "form in which the food is served is to be that to which the men are accustomed." While the soldier could be given a ration of bread, bacon, and beans, Richards claimed, the Harvard boat crew required some "frills," such as ice cream and strawberry shortcake.[113]

Dietary advice protected the distinctions of class with particular vigilance in places where social mingling threatened to obscure social boundaries and hierarchies. The constant intermingling of the classes that resulted from urbanization and industrialization presented challenges to maintaining the distinct identity and status of the middle class.[114] In *The Cost of Food* Richards provided rules for eating in the kinds of places where people from different class backgrounds inevitably mixed, such as hospitals, penal institutions, and households with maids. She argued that in hospitals, for example, the different grades of employees should be given different diets that accurately reflected their income, occupation, and habituated preferences. In large hospitals, she explained, the four grades of employees (house officers and heads of departments; nurses and second assistants; engineers and workmen; scrubwomen, janitors, and choremen) should be fed in separate rooms with different hours, menus, and costs.[115] Economy was typically Richards's foremost priority, but she was so concerned about keeping the diets of each group of workers separate that she advised spending more to do so. The same was true for patients, whose diets, she felt, should not be changed by a stay in the hospital. For those with "cultivated tastes," no expense was to be spared in providing the finest food, but for those "for whom corned beef and cabbage represents a luxury," Richards advised, "it is not necessary to stimulate an artificial appetite." While cream, fruit, and other delicacies should be available for paying patients, as well as for doctors and nurses, Richards advised that attendants and other "hearty" workers be forbidden to taste them. She went so far as to suggest that such foods should be kept under lock and key, if necessary, to prevent infractions against the class-based dietary order.[116]

The advice about eating right that domestic scientists gave American women at the turn of the century reflected a nuanced understanding of the constituent aspects of class and attempted to secure the boundaries of the nascent middle class through a number of strategies that constructed dietary distinctions. These strategies naturalized the differences between the healthy middle class and the unhealthy other, between brain workers and manual workers, between members of the Harvard boat crew and soldiers in the field, which were in fact cultural. They imputed a biological component to class by conflating the physiological and the environmental components of dietary health.[117] As the middle class made health a foundation of its character and identity, domestic science provided the dietary beliefs and practices that would also secure the viability of the class, in theory at least, through eating right.

ELLEN RICHARDS passionately championed the social role lessons in eating right might play in the making of a new America held together by a shared set of irrefutable principles, oriented around a commitment to the social good, and populated by good citizens whose domestic habits reinforced the values of Progressivism. In her brazen embrace of lessons in natural law as a way to curb freedom and chasten those who would resist the interventions of government on behalf of the greater good, those of us living a century later can see clearly the links between dietary reform and social reform, dietary ideals and social ideals, that are still with us, although they have become increasingly difficult to discern. Home economists embraced first moral uplift and then citizen training as the aim of dietary reform because to them the dual function of dietary ideals—both as rules about what to eat and as a means of self-making—was self-evident. A century later, scientific nutritional ideals are taken for granted. The basic principles of scientific nutrition were common knowledge by the end of World War I, and though the science has continuously evolved to incorporate new findings and respond to new social concerns, nutrition has remained the prevailing mode of thinking about food value and dietary health. But science has come to be perceived as distinct from values, politics, and morals, which obscures the social content embedded in dietary ideals and the social role played by dietary reform.[118]

The critic Gyorgy Scrinis refers to the prevailing mode of thinking about food in terms of its nutrient content as the "ideology or paradigm of *nutritionism*." He argues that nutritionism is naturalized through the workings of nutrition scientists, dieticians, public-health practitioners, and the food industry, and that it eclipses other modes of understanding and assessing the value of food, such as level of processing, means of agricultural production, sensual properties, and cultural or historical significance.[119] But even this trenchant critique, which was popularized by Michael Pollan in his bestselling book *In Defense of Food*, overlooks the ideological work of nutrition that the story of Wilbur Atwater, Ellen Richards, and domestic science reveals.[120] Their story shows that nutrition is more than just a way of assessing food value, or even delimiting what counts as food value. It's an ideology that governs not just how we think about food, but also how we think about ourselves and other people. Nutrition provides guidelines about how to be a good person and a good citizen, a means of self-making, and a quantifiable moral measure that can be used to assess and compare others. Their story also shows that nutrition and the American middle class emerged together in part through a mutually constitutive process that depended on the construction of a dangerously "unhealthy other." It reminds us that there is no such thing as dietary health apart from social ideals and that dietary assessment is inseparable from a moral hierarchy that is inevitably classed. But their story is just the beginning of the history of modern American dietary reform. In the century or so that followed, while the definitions of both a good diet and a good citizen continued to evolve, dietary advice maintained its ethical function, providing lessons in eating right that connected diet and citizenship. Meanwhile, the scope and purview of dietary reform grew. The first of two major expansions in the overall reach and significance of dietary discourse took place during World War II, as nutritional concerns converged with social anxieties and aspirations to make eating right a wartime duty for every American.

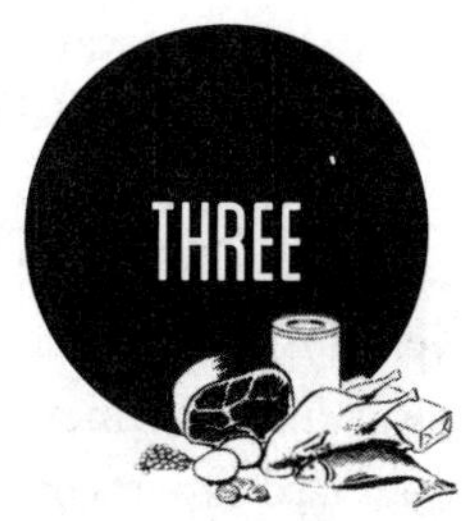

ANXIETY AND ASPIRATION ON THE NUTRITION FRONT

At the height of the mobilization for World War II, President Roosevelt called a three-day conference to address nutrition as a defense problem. Presiding over the conference, Paul McNutt opened with a resounding call for action that captured the urgency and gravitas that impending war brought to dietary health in both its empirical and its ethical aspects. "This," he announced, "is a call to save the American way of life by making it possible for every single person—at every place on the income scale—to achieve maximum health and vigor by alleviating both hollow hunger (of those who have not enough food) and hidden hunger (of those who are malnourished due to ignorance).... Good nutrition can make people who seem unproductive or like trouble makers into good, productive members of society." McNutt, who had recently been appointed administrator of the Federal Security Agency and coordinator of Health, Welfare, and Related Defense Activities, went on to explain to the nine hundred invited delegates in attendance that they had been brought together to discuss nutrition for two reasons.[1] One was clearly connected to the empirical aspects of nutrition, which had undergone a significant change since the domestic-science era: "First, new and startling facts about nutrition have become known—facts which are vital to the strength, health, and security of the United States." The other made clear the social importance those nutritional facts had suddenly attained as the nation prepared for war: "Second, the Unites States faces today one of the greatest crises in its history—a crisis of such broad significance that we cannot afford to compromise our national strength in any way. If we lose, our way of life will fall, perhaps forever."[2]

Precisely because it provided both a set of rules for how to eat right *and* a means of self-making, nutrition became central to the wartime demand for a vigorous, capable, and willing population. Combined with new discoveries about the role of vitamins, the war set into motion a major expansion in the scope and significance of dietary reform. In the hands of wartime reformers—not crusading activists but federally mandated, recognized experts in nutrition, food, and health—eating right was reframed as a social duty for every single American. Driven by both profound anxieties about the dangers of bad diets and unfettered optimism about what could be possible if eating habits were improved, wartime dietary reformers set out to ensure morale, productivity, and victory by teaching Americans on the home front to eat right.

From an Invisible Epidemic to the Fittest Nation the World Has Ever Seen

The discovery of vitamins between 1910 and 1920 undermined the logic of early nutrition and set into motion a paradigmatic shift in dietary ideals that would eventually converge with social concerns related to the World War II mobilization. Prior to that, however, the dietary ideals that Atwater and domestic scientists promoted were thrust into the national consciousness by efforts during World War I to reduce food waste and minimize the use of foods made scarce by the war. The Food Administration drew on Atwater's findings that energy sources were interchangeable, urging the substitution of popular but scarce foods such as meat, flour, and butter with nutritionally similar but more available ones like beans, oats, and lard.[3] By the end of the First World War, millions of people had learned "that there were things called calories, and that some foods were similar to each other and others were not."[4] But the discovery of vitamins complicated the "pecuniary economy of food" and caused the nutrition community to rethink whether or not Americans were well fed. The transition began with the biochemist Elmer McCollum's experiments on rats, which in 1908 proved there was an element of food essential for life and health that had not been detected in Atwater's work with human subjects. In 1911

Casimir Funk managed to isolate one of these nutrients, and by 1912 McCollum had isolated another and linked its absence to vision and growth problems in rats. In 1916 he proved a direct link between the absence of vitamin B and the human disease beriberi. In the course of the next ten years, a stream of discoveries about the importance of vitamins, as well as of minerals and trace elements, transformed the American concept of an adequate diet.[5] By the early 1920s, a new way of thinking about a good diet, which McCollum called "the newer knowledge of nutrition," was sweeping the nation. Food marketers helped to popularize the new nutritional paradigm; desperate for ways to differentiate their products, they used vitamin-related health claims to tout everything from Fleischmann's Yeast ("the richest known source of soluble vitamins"), to Welch's grape juice ("Rich in Health Values") and Morton's Salt ("Health Salt").[6]

The discovery of vitamins may have been good for business, but it overturned existing understandings of the relationship between diet and health, producing both a sense of uneasiness that bad eating habits might be more dangerous than nutritionists had thought and optimism about what vitamins could do for health and longevity. The links between vitamins and deficiency diseases raised the specter that people who seemed to be eating right under the reign of the caloric paradigm might actually be consuming too few vitamin-rich "protective foods" and, therefore, be missing important elements in their diets. Meanwhile, experiments showed that the *presence* of vitamins not only protected against deficiency diseases but also had the potential to enhance health, increase vitality, and improve longevity, which led to hopes that good diets could create new levels of physical and national well-being. The threat and promise of vitamins mirrored the uncertainty and ambition that accompanied the transition from a massive economic depression to the demands of mobilization. This alchemy of nutritional and social anxieties and aspirations resulted in an expansion of the reach of dietary reform across the entire population and, as eating right became a problem for every American, lessons in eating right were positioned to play an important ideological role on the home front and beyond.

The discovery of vitamins produced uneasiness about the nutritional welfare of the nation because it upset established knowledge and raised fears the nutrition community did not yet have the tools to allay. The discovery of the link between vitamins and deficiency diseases complicated the central tenet of germ theory, that disease was caused by foreign elements entering the system, and utterly undermined the central logic of the caloric system, that the efficient production of energy was the sole aim of nutrition. As an article in the *New York Times* put it, "When it was discovered that a man might gorge himself on calories and yet starve to death, our conception of a good diet changed."[7] Clearly, vitamins were essential, but there was no way to assess whether or not people were getting enough of them. There was no standard for how much of any given vitamin people needed to consume, no consensus on the vitamin content of various foods, and no established method of measuring the adequacy of individual diets within the new paradigm. Because the effects of vitamin deficiency, short of full-blown deficiency diseases, were more or less invisible, nutrition experts armed with this new but incomplete knowledge began to suspect that people who appeared perfectly healthy might actually be suffering from subtle yet serious nutritional deficiencies. The fact that vitamins were invisible, odorless, and tasteless added to their mystique (and their allure) and fueled anxiety that diets previously thought to be adequate might in fact be dangerously lacking, and people who appeared to be well might actually be malnourished.

Depression-era nutrition studies appeared to confirm the worst fears of nutritionists who suspected that Americans were not consuming enough protective foods. In the mid-1930s home economists working under federal auspices set out to see how well the diets of American families were faring in the Depression. Because there were no established norms and methods for assessing nutritional well-being, however, the researchers were forced to improvise. Not surprisingly, they devised studies that confirmed their preconceptions about how financial hardship combined with ignorance about the importance of "protective foods" were undermining the health of the population. One approach commonly used by researchers involved measuring a household's food expenditures in order to determine whether or not family members were getting enough of the essential nutrients. In a reversal of the logic of Atwater's era, researchers assumed that the more money families spent on food, the better their diets were.[8] Families with constrained food budgets were automatically considered poorly nourished. Other studies used notoriously inaccurate recall surveys along with rough estimates of dietary needs to determine nutritional status. For example, the USDA home economist Hazel Stiebeling asked families to recall what they had eaten over the course of a week, then estimated the amount of nutrition this would have supplied. She labeled diets poor if they failed to meet the estimated requirement for one or more of the nutrients considered essential, which included but was not limited to protein, calcium, phosphorous, iron, vitamin A, thiamin, riboflavin, and ascorbic acid.[9] Not surprisingly, more than a third of American families were found to have only fair diets and another third or more were found to be consuming diets considered poor.[10] Stiebeling's findings were not taken lightly; they led President Roosevelt to declare one-third of the nation "ill-nourished" in his 1937 inaugural address.[11]

The kind of malnutrition that so worried researchers during the late 1930s and early 1940s was not "hollow hunger," caused by not having enough food, but what came to be known as "hidden hunger." Invented in the late 1930s, the diagnosis "hidden hunger" captured the intertwined nutritional and social anxieties of the era.[12] If hollow hunger was a caloric deficiency caused by the inability to attain adequate quantities of food, hidden hunger reflected the more complicated nutritional paradigm that had been ushered in by the discovery of vitamins. Hollow hunger was evident in the ravaged bodies and acute suffering of the underfed, but the effects of hidden hunger were less obvious, more subtle. Caused by failure to choose the right kinds of foods, hidden hunger was believed to take its toll in the form of fatigue, aches and pains, digestive problems, and lowered disease resistance. Its "danger signals" were a vague compendium of ill-defined symptoms that had no proven link to diet but were nonetheless attributed to poor eating habits: underweight and overweight, poor posture, flabby muscles, lack of strength, lack of energy, tiring easily, lack of mental alertness, depression, feeling cross and fussy.[13] A defining characteristic of hidden hunger was that it was nearly impossible to detect. Even the medical establishment seemed unable to document its impact; while dietary studies convinced researchers that the affliction was frighteningly pervasive, physicians found no evidence of widespread malnutrition among the population.[14] But the fact that evidence of malnutrition was hard to come by only inflamed anxieties about a dietary threat that was both pernicious and elusive.

In evoking a vaguely defined, ever-present, but nearly undetectable threat, the concept of hidden hunger expressed anxieties that attended the transition from the Depression to the mobilization for war and set into motion a historic expansion in the scope and purview of dietary reform. The concept of hidden hunger extended concerns about eating habits that had emerged from Depression-era research beyond the population whose diets were limited by financial hardship to all Americans who might, unknowingly, be consuming inadequate diets. As McNutt explained at the National Nutrition Conference for Defense, hidden hunger was caused by people "filling up on bad things because they don't know any better."[15] It shifted concern from access to adequate food among the poor, a thorny political matter during the Depression, to nutrition education for the entire population, an aim that resonated well with the social politics of the home front.[16] Hidden hunger broadened the scope of dietary reform, transforming hunger from a poor person's problem to a threat to national well-being that demanded population-wide interventions.

The threat of war turned hidden hunger into a national-defense issue and dietary reform—for the entire population—into a home-front priority. As the nation began mobilizing for war in 1940, hidden hunger expressed and reflected growing fears about whether or not American men, having just endured a long Depression, were up to the task of fighting for their country. By September 1940, France had fallen to the Nazis and the rest of Europe was in danger of doing the same. Hitler was attacking British air defenses and an invasion across the English Channel seemed imminent. Meanwhile, the Selective Service Committee announced that 380,000 of the first million men called for service had been rejected on medical grounds. One observer remarked that revelations about the condition of young men were handled with optimism at first, but "as the underweight and the overweight, as young men with half their teeth gone, as the flabby and the generally run-down appeared before the examiners, an uneasy feeling developed."[17] The widely reported rejections were based on a broad range of conditions, including poor teeth; eye, cardiovascular, nervous, and mental conditions; underweight and overweight; and gonorrhea and syphilis.[18] There was no clear evidence directly linking any of these ailments to diet, but the concept of hidden hunger provided a ready alibi. The deputy director of the Selective Service System, Lewis B. Hershey, blamed eating habits for at least a third of the rejections. He conceded that it was not his job to "fix causes for these disabilities," but nonetheless went on to say, "Foods undoubtedly play a very considerable part, whether it be because of lack of proper amount, or because the food was of an improper kind."[19] Two hundred thousand of the unfit were deemed capable of "limited military service," and another hundred thousand were deemed "capable of rehabilitation to the point where they can do full military service," which left only eighty thousand rejected and only a third of those for causes believed but not known to be nutrition related, but these facts were buried in the anxiety and excitement.[20] With the Selective Service rejections, hidden hunger, an expression of interlinked nutritional and social concerns, officially became a defense issue.

In the fall of 1940 President Roosevelt gave the National Defense Council approval to designate Paul V. McNutt "coordinator of all health, medical, welfare, nutrition, recreation and other related fields of activity affecting the national defense."[21] At the same time, the National Research Council was asked to establish an advisory group to assist in wartime food policy. In response it set up two boards: the Food and Nutrition Board (FNB) was designed to explore the biochemical and physiological side of nutrition, and the Committee on Food Habits (CFH) was intended to study food consumption and attitudes toward food from a cultural standpoint. When the president charged McNutt with the task of improving the nation's nutrition status, McNutt's first step was to ask the FNB to figure out how much of each nutrient was needed for good health; it was time to establish a quantifiable measure for dietary health that fit "the newer knowledge of nutrition." In response to this request, the head of the FNB gave three home economists until the following morning to come up with a standard recommendation of nutrients based on existing research. Not surprisingly, they reported that it could not be done because the "evidence was too scanty and conflicting."[22] A committee formed under the direction of one of the women spent the next year reviewing existing research and seeking consensus within the nutrition community, a process that ultimately resulted in the nation's first Recommended Dietary Allowances (RDAS).[23]

On the empirical level, the RDAS were the dietary standards that researchers and reformers needed in order to assess and improve eating habits. But where hidden hunger built on the invisible dangers of vitamin deficiency to express anxiety about the well-being of the nation, the RDAS capitalized on the somewhat magical promise of vitamin consumption to both legitimate the need for nutrition reform and express an unbounded sense of national ambition. While the invisible danger of vitamin deficiency extended the possibility of malnutrition indefinitely, the potential of vitamin abundance did the same for the possibility of dietary health. The RDAS were meant to be estimates because, as the committee that devised them noted, there was a "lack of sufficient experimental evidence on which to base estimated requirements for the various nutrients with any great degree of accuracy."[24] At the same time, they were designed to instill the idea that every American needed to strive for better eating habits, improved health, and more vigor.[25]

The RDAS, which were formally announced on a coast-to-coast radio broadcast on the eve of the opening of the National Nutrition Conference for Defense, did not aim simply for adequate diets. Instead of choosing standards that reflected the average of expert recommendations, the committee, after some debate, agreed to include a "margin of safety" of almost 30 percent.[26] Those who had advocated lower limits were appeased by the use of the term *allowances*, rather than *standards*, but adequacy was never the aim. As the professor of nutrition Henry Sherman explained at the National Nutrition Conference for Defense, "Improvement in this direction does not stop at adequacy. . . . There may be and often are very important differences between the merely adequate and the optimal in nutrition. Better growth and development, higher attainment in stamina and working efficiency, and a longer lease of healthier and more useful life, may all be realized in the same individuals through the fuller use of the newest knowledge of nutrition."[27] Also speaking at the conference, Vice President Henry Wallace described the long-term goals as not only to wipe out deficiency diseases and reduce the rate of negative health effects caused by poor diets, but also to seek, for everyone in the United States, the feeling of "health-plus."[28] For members of the FNB, the margin of safety was a key part of an ambitious plan for optimum nutrition. The board's 1943 report soundly rejected the notion, proposed by critics, that people who failed to meet the margin of safety were not deficient; according to a Harvard nutritionist, the RDAS were set so high that "nearly everyone in the population can consume less than the standard yet be adequately nourished."[29] On the contrary, the FNB argued that optimum nutrition levels should be the aim of the nutrition program and that anything less should be considered insufficient. The report explained, "As far as the immediate or long term well-being of a person can be improved through dietary betterment, that person falls short of being truly well fed."[30]

The ambitious RDAS had the immediate effects of exacerbating concerns about American eating habits and of expanding the purview of reform by reframing dietary health as a problem that every single American needed to be concerned about. When researchers reviewed the dietary studies of the mid-1930s using the new standards, they determined that those already alarming results were actually too "optimistic" and systematically downgraded the previous assessment. A subcommittee of the FNB worried, for example, that in the earlier studies, the use of the term *fair* was probably misleading, since people might think the diet labeled "fair" had "a certain degree of goodness." In fact, the committee explained, "fair" represented "a degree of inferiority. . . . A diet that falls short, even so slightly, and permits development of deficiency states may be relatively fair but it is absolutely unsafe." Diets that had once been deemed fair, they argued, should be viewed as "unsatisfactory" and those diets once labeled "poor" should be regarded as "very poor."[31] The FNB also argued for a widespread reappraisal of American dietary health; bodily states previously regarded as healthy were to be reclassified as pathological. They began to use the term *latent malnutrition* to describe the slow, subtle, and barely detectable forms of dietary deficiency threatening the population, and explained that physicians were not finding signs of widespread malnutrition across the population because they had been trained to detect only acute manifestations. The real threat, however, came from the long, slow process of chronic malnutrition caused by bad diets over many years.[32] The committee warned, "So common, so prevalent, so frequently seen are some of these changes, especially their slighter degrees, that they have been regarded as usual or normal."[33] The medical community, the committee went on to argue, needed to learn to recognize that states of health previously considered normal were in fact dangerous deficiency states.[34]

These new understandings of dietary danger, dietary promise, and the need for every American to eat right were echoed throughout the National Nutrition Conference for Defense. Speeches captured the core sentiments of the new era of dietary reform: that malnutrition was everywhere yet nearly impossible to detect, that eating right could lead to new heights of health and strength, and that it was therefore the duty of every American to strive for better eating habits. The surgeon general issued this ominous warning: "Like an iceberg, nine-tenths of our malnutrition, and the most dangerous part, is under the surface."[35] The chairman of the Nutrition Advisory Committee, M. L. Wilson, made it clear that the era of hollow hunger, in which only the poor suffered malnutrition, was over. Science, he explained, "uncovered starvation in places where it was not supposed to exist, in high and middle places as well as in the low." Starvation was no longer a matter of not having enough food, but rather a problem of failing to choose the right kinds of foods: "Call it malnutrition, call it undernourishment, call it dietary deficiency, or what you will—when men and women and children fail to eat the foods that give them full life and vigor, they are in fact starving."[36]

Speakers also celebrated the new heights of national strength and vitality that could result from every citizen striving to eat right. While dietary improvement was necessary because at least a third of the population was suffering from ill health due to poor eating habits, it was perhaps even more important because eating right could improve the health of people who were already well. As Henry Sherman explained, "The first of these aspects is clearly an urgent essential of national defense, and an obvious duty to our fellow citizens. The second aspect can mean an advance of even more far-reaching significance."[37] In his closing remarks, Surgeon General Thomas Parran also expressed the expansive dietary ambition behind wartime dietary reform, declaring that the nutrition program had the potential to build "a nation of people more fit, more vigorous, more competent; a nation with better morale, a more unified purpose, more toughness of body, and greater strength of mind that the world has ever seen." He referred to "the building up of our own people to a level of health and vigor never before attained or even dreamed of," and ended the conference by declaring that nutrition reform could build "a new, a stronger, a more intelligent, a more competent race. Yes, food will build a new America."[38]

Changing Food Habits, Making Wartime Citizens

The new nutritional truths—that every American might be quietly suffering from hidden hunger and that few diets met the requirements of optimum nutrition laid out by the RDAS—extended the scope of dietary reform to include every citizen, just as the context of total war demanded home-front programs that could help boost morale. As many historians have argued, home-front campaigns such as bond drives and scrap collections had ideological aims that may have been even more important than their material ones. They promoted nationalism and supported morale by channeling civilian energies into tasks that were given meaning through promotional propaganda.[39] Among these home-front campaigns were several distinct but coordinated efforts to manage the food supply and keep both soldiers and civilians well fed during the war. While food programs that encouraged rationing, conservation, and the production and preservation of food through victory gardens and canning have been recognized as having played an important social role on the home front, we know less about the role played by the National Nutrition Program, a home-front dietary reform movement that focused on nutrition education.[40] Wartime dietary reformers—experts from across the professional spectrum working at the federal, state, and local levels—connected good diets to good morale and good wartime citizenship, building on the dual nature of dietary ideals to provide rules about what to eat that also functioned as a means of self-making. Like home-economics courses that were designed to help people to adjust to the demands of Progressive Era citizenship, wartime lessons in eating right both promoted the new dietary standards and helped people to adjust to the exigencies of wartime citizenship.

Many home-front programs had both material and social aims, but the nature of food made it an especially appealing tool for wartime propaganda. The Office of War Information (OWI), responsible for propaganda campaigns, asserted that food presented a unique and especially powerful means of orienting citizens toward the war effort. Its "Food Fights for Freedom" campaign was explicitly intended to capitalize on the intimate role of food in people's daily routines and social lives. With the aim of turning food into "the deadliest weapon of all," the program provided information about the challenges facing the food supply as rations were shipped abroad and production facilities focused on defense needs, and it outlined the actions that civilians were expected to take to ease shortages and maintain the levels of health and vigor demanded by total war. In advising the media on how to present information about food to the public in 1943, the OWI noted that food might not inspire the same kind of motivation as cooperative efforts aimed at producing more battleships and bombers, but argued that the "personal appeal" of food in the lives of individuals gave it a powerful resonance and a unique advantage on which the campaign for home-front morale should capitalize.[41] Food was particularly well suited to the job of enlisting Americans in the war effort because it was "a keystone of the home" and a focal point for social occasions. Sharing food created fellowship, and food had a unique emotional appeal that could be leveraged in the interest of the war effort. "The language of food is universal," the OWI explained. "A whole galaxy of human emotions revolve around the stark fact that man must eat to live. These emotions provide an inexhaustible source of appeals for action."[42] Just as they were buying war bonds and saving rubber and fat, the OWI declared, every citizen needed to learn to think of food as "not just a means of selfish satisfaction, but as a crucial, vital war material. In our hearts we can learn to rank food in importance with bonds, machine tools, rubber and waste fat—with guns, tanks, ships, planes."[43] Under the umbrella of the Food Fights for Freedom program, "appeals for action" included urging people to produce foods in victory gardens, conserve through canning and proper cooking techniques, adjust diets to availability, observe rationing and price ceilings, and practice good nutrition.

The food program was shaped by a tension common to the home-front programs: the fight against totalitarianism fueled a celebration of democracy—some have argued democracy was elevated to the status of a "civil religion"—while it also demanded new levels of social control.[44] The aim of the food program was to manage the eating habits of the population in the best interests of the war effort, but it was critical that the principles of democracy be preserved, not compromised, in the process. Speaking at the National Nutrition Conference for Defense, Harriet Elliot, assistant administrator in charge of the Consumer Division, Office of Price Administration, explained the need for an approach that would strengthen, not undermine, democracy in the process of defending it. "Defense cannot be wholly for the people," she argued, "it must be by the people."[45] These concerns about democracy were evident in the way the nutrition program was designed, executed, and represented. While the nutrition program was directed by the federal government, it was meant to be carried out by citizens working in their own communities. As M. L. Wilson, head of the Nutrition and Food Conservation branch of the War Food Administration explained, the nutrition program was intended to advance democratic ideals through a structure that emphasized the input and involvement of every citizen. In his foreword to *Democracy Means All of Us*, a manual designed to help communities organize wartime nutrition programs, Wilson celebrated the fact that the nutrition program worked through a network of channels rather than as a "hierarchy of power groups." He hailed nutrition as a way that "all of our 130,000,000 people, working through local, state, regional, and national nutrition committees" could actively practice democracy. He wrote, "Thousands of Americans see in the nutrition program an opportunity to take the kind of responsibility for public action which is part and parcel of the democratic tradition."[46]

In keeping with these ideals, the nutrition campaign was directed and coordinated at the federal level through the nutrition division of the Office of Defense Health and Welfare Services (ODHWS), but it was implemented throughout the country by state and local nutrition committees.[47] State nutrition committees were composed of representatives of federal agencies including the Bureau of Home Economics, the Children's Bureau, the Extension Service, the Farm Security Administration, and the Public Health Service. They also included representatives from state-level organizations such as colleges, boards of education, state departments, and health departments. Private and local organizations—including medical, dental, dietetics, and home-economics associations, the American Red Cross, farm organizations, public schools, "racial group" organizations, and private health and welfare agencies—also had representatives.[48] State nutrition committees functioned as steering committees and clearinghouses for information and plans, but the real action took place at the local level. Representatives from civic, educational, professional, social, religious, youth, and commercial groups served on the local committees and took on the task of making their communities "aware of the importance of nutrition in relation to health."[49] They used a wide range of activities to reach their neighbors. They formed discussion groups, study groups, and reading lists, established information and consultation centers, produced regular press releases and radio programs, and staged special campaigns such as "nutrition weeks." They also placed exhibits in store windows, libraries, schools, and other public places, and planned food demonstrations and gardening and home-production programs.[50] Local committees often prepared their own educational materials, but also received reference, educational, and promotional materials—from posters to radio scripts—from the ODHWS and the state committees.

From the state and local nutrition committees operating across the country came lessons in eating right that capitalized on both the empirical and the ethical aspects of nutrition. The central nutritional guidelines of the program, the "Basic 7" food guide, clearly operated on both of these levels (see figure 3.1). The practical aim of the Basic 7 was to increase the consumption of vitamin-rich or "protective foods" by teaching people to choose foods from each of seven categories every day. On the em-

For Health...eat some food
from each group...every day!
GROUP ONE
GREEN AND YELLOW
VEGETABLES...
some raw—some cooked,
frozen or canned
GROUP TWO
ORANGES, TOMATOES,
GRAPEFRUIT...
or raw cabbage or salad greens
GROUP THREE
POTATOES AND OTHER
VEGETABLES AND FRUITS
raw, dried, cooked,
frozen or canned
GROUP FOUR
MILK AND
MILK PRODUCTS...
fluid, evaporated,
dried milk, or cheese
GROUP FIVE
MEAT, POULTRY,
FISH, OR EGGS...
or dried beans, peas,
nuts, or peanut butter
GROUP SIX
GROUP SEVEN
BUTTER AND
FORTIFIED MARGARINE
(with added Vitamin A)
U.S. NEEDS US STRONG
EAT THE BASIC 7 EVERY DAY
U.S. GOVERNMENT CHART
IN ADDITION TO THE BASIC 7...
EAT ANY OTHER FOODS YOU WANT
U S DEPARTMENT OF AGRICULTURE

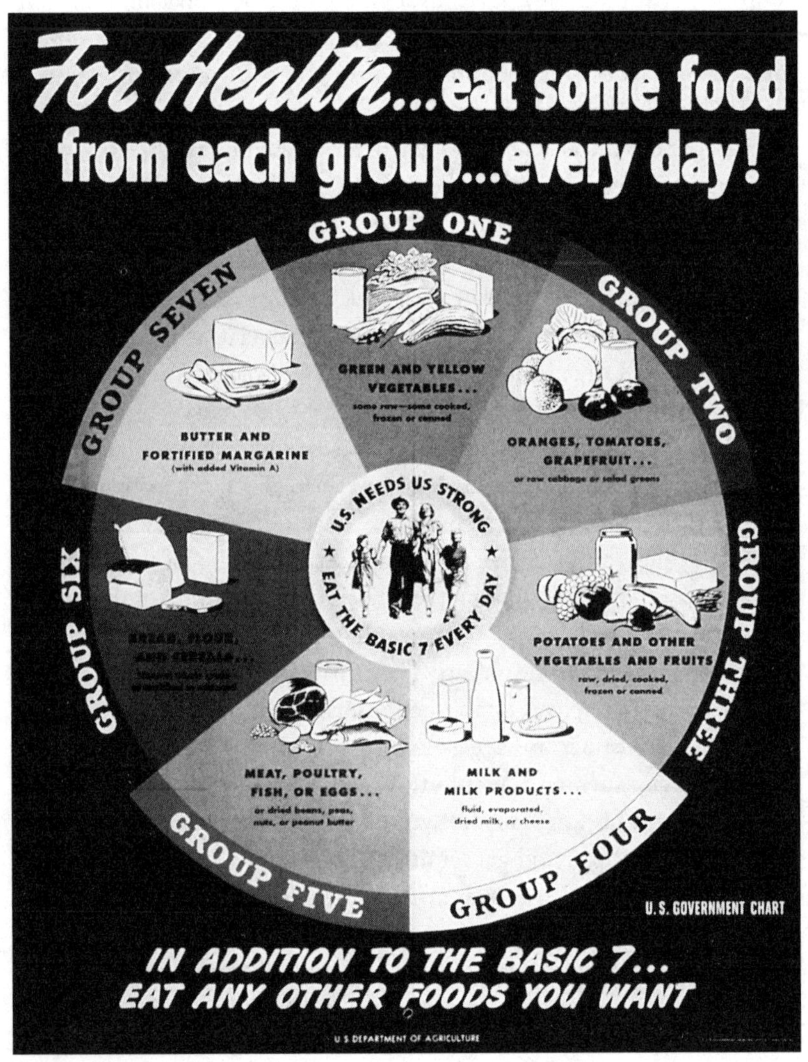

FIGURE 3.1 • Empirical meets ethical on the home front. Courtesy of National Archives, photo 44-PA-798B.

pirical level, the Basic 7 translated the highly technical RDAS into simple advice that people could relate to and follow in choosing what to eat. At the same time, it leveraged the self-making function of dietary ideals by presenting eating right as a means through which individuals could align their daily habits with the war effort and practice good wartime citizenship. The guide was usually presented as a circle divided into seven segments representing groups of nutritionally similar foods from which people were supposed to eat every day: green and yellow vegetables; oranges, tomatoes, grapefruit; potatoes and other vegetables and fruit; milk and milk products; meat, poultry, fish, and eggs; bread, flour, and cereals; butter and fortified margarine. In addition to displaying a graphic lesson in choosing a varied diet, the guide also provided a visual depiction of the social significance of eating right: a typical representation of the Basic 7 also included an image in the center—in red, white, and blue—of a family of four walking toward the viewer. The image was framed by the motto "U.S. Needs Us Strong: Eat the Basic 7 Every Day." The picture of the stalwart family facing the future together, brave and unified, made it clear that "U.S. Needs Us Strong" referred not only to the imperative for physical strength during wartime, but also to the equally important need for social stability and cohesion. Together, the dietary guidelines, the motto, and the image of the family suggested that eating right was a patriotic wartime duty central to the pursuit of both of these aims.

The idea that good diets were somehow linked to that intangible sense of unity of purpose and confidence in a shared goal known as morale was often made explicit. For example, the pamphlet *Feeding Four on a Dollar a Day*—originally produced in Denver and so popular that it was eventually made into a radio show—explained that knowledge of nutrition had become a "patriotic duty for everyone" that would "pay dividends in family, health and life, and national strength." It listed three reasons why it was essential to study nutrition during the war: "Food can win or lose the war" (the use of food as a military tactic); "food can 'make or break' our nation" (the use of food to ensure the "health and strength" of the population); and "food can build or destroy morale" (the "knowledge of nutrition" as "a patriotic duty for everyone today"). The pamphlet described vitamins as essential for morale and made a direct connection between eating right and having a good attitude about the war: "It may be that our 'sour puss' friends are suffering from some form of malnutrition! It is an established fact that family morale, war morale is closely knit to the food we eat."[51]

The idea that choosing the right foods was an essential component of a stable and cooperative home front was embedded in wartime dietary lessons even when the concept of morale itself was not explicitly used. Throughout the pamphlets, posters, plays, radio briefs, lectures, and other wartime nutrition-education materials, eating right was equated with the physical and social qualities that were considered essential for good wartime citizenship, from stamina to courage and cooperativeness. A robust nutrition program in New York State that was guided by home economists at Cornell University left behind a wealth of materials that both reveal the extent of the nutrition effort and show how dietary reform functioned as a pedagogy of good wartime citizenship. In 1941 alone, the College of Home Economics at Cornell distributed over 52,000 bulletins and leaflets, broadcast over 300 radio talks, led roughly 8,600 local leader training meetings, made almost 17,000 phone calls, and conducted about 5,000 demonstrations. A report on activities between 1941 and 1942 documented that almost 168,000 people had attended local leader training meetings and estimated that over 24,000 families were reporting "better balanced meals" as a result of their efforts.[52] Yet "better balanced meals" were but one component of what the reformers were out to accomplish.

The efforts of the New York State Nutrition Committee, like those of other state and local nutrition committees, were geared toward conveying both the empirical and the ethical aspects of eating right. They taught the facts of "newer nutrition," promoted wartime social ideals, and depicted a direct relationship between good diets and good wartime citizenship. Radio briefs read on the state's airwaves, for example, taught listeners that eating right was central to the overall mission of victory, and that diets were key to both the physiological and the mental aspects of being a good wartime citizen. In "Your Child's Eating Habits" the announcer declared, "Nutrition scientists go so far as to say that a poor diet may be the cause of lack of courage and willpower. And that is a matter of importance in these emergency times. The country needs to have every citizen physically and mentally fit to take part in the big job of defense. So you can do a great favor not only to your child but also to your country by guiding him in the food habits that build health and character."[53] "Food First," another radio brief, also taught that nutrition was essential for reasons that went beyond the physiological: "Courage, cooperativeness, and productive capacity—as well as the good old-fashioned feeling of buoyant and good health—are all very important to national defense. And they all depend upon proper food."[54] The New York State Nutrition Committee also published a pamphlet that described people who ate a good diet as "more apt to be alert, energetic, optimistic, cooperative; they are more apt to have clear eyes, good eyesight at night, good muscles, good posture, good color, straight, strong bones, and a sense of well-being." The same pamphlet declared, "For the all-out effort of the defense program, we need people who are physically fit and capable of sustained effort and boundless enthusiasm in order to accomplish the gigantic task ahead for victory: victory in the battle for good nutrition as well as in the battle of production."[55]

Nutrition educators leveraged the ethical aspects of dietary ideals not only by conflating the features of good nutrition and good citizenship, but also by quite literally engaging people in the process of nutritional self-improvement as a wartime civic duty. Means for measuring oneself against the nutritional norm of the RDAs proliferated throughout the war years. Scorecards, checklists, and other devices for self-assessment made it possible for people to see exactly how far their eating habits fell from the ideal and encouraged them to practice nutritional self-improvement in the name of victory. For example, a "Personal Nutrition Record" provided by General Mills for use in nutrition study groups encouraged people to assess their eating habits against the Basic 7, then sign a pledge promising to improve them. In signing the pledge, the participant promised to "establish good food habits and follow them, knowing that by building a healthy body and strong nerves I can get more out of life myself and do more for others. I'll be proud, too, of being a strong American."[56]

A nutrition course developed at Cornell for 4-H clubs demonstrates exactly how reformers imagined nutritional self-assessment could lead to self-improvement and self-making geared toward becoming a good citizen. The aim of the course, called "What Foods to Eat and Why," was not only to teach the tenets of nutrition, but also to engage the students in a process of self-making through nutritional self-improvement. The students learned the fundamentals of nutrition by studying charts, preparing foods rich in vitamin A, making lists of calcium- and iron-rich foods, and comparing the nutritional contributions of eggs, milk, cake, and lettuce. But they also learned to think about following the rules of nutrition in terms of the kind of person they would become as they learned to eat right.

The first meeting was called, "A Well Nourished Person Is Strong and Capable." It taught the "relation between the appearance, size and condition of a person and the care with which he eats," and enlisted students in the process of improving their own habits. Students filled out "How Well Do I Eat?" cards and listed the exact corrections that his or her diet needed. For the next meeting each student prepared a report on "how his food habits are going to be improved," and a progress report was required at each subsequent meeting. The second meeting emphasized the "relation between the fine appearance, the pep and the kindliness of men and women and the care with which they eat." The next taught the relation of food to physical factors (appearance, endurance, nervous and muscular control) and mental factors (alertness, vitality, emotional stability, and disposition). The fourth meeting, called "A Well Nourished Person Can Choose His Way and Travel It," made a strong case for learning to eat right in order to be a good citizen by comparing "the possibilities for building a busy, useful, eventful and happy life of a poorly nourished boy or girl with that of a well-nourished one."[57]

While wartime reformers approached teaching people to eat right as a process that could shape good citizens, they were concerned that it also had the dangerous potential of misshaping them—a possibility about which the members of the Committee on Food Habits worried explicitly. The mandate of the CFH, which worked alongside the FNB, was to figure out how to get people to eat in accordance with scientific knowledge or, as they put it, to determine "the most effective ways and means of adjusting habit to needs, of getting people to wish what they need."[58] But the committee was made up of anthropologists and other social scientists who were extremely sensitive to the inevitable social impact of changing people's eating habits. By 1942, the members had become concerned that efforts to "bring dietary habits into conformity with dietary needs" might be fundamentally at odds with the concepts of choice and freedom that were so fundamental to democracy, and that if they followed through on such a mandate they were likely to produce citizens who were better prepared for life in a totalitarian society.[59] In a 1942 report published in the *Journal of Home Economics*, for example, committee member Mary Sweeny explained that the committee felt that extolling a person to give up bad food habits for good ones was "tantamount to asking him to undertake to fetter himself with a set of good chains in place of a set of bad chains." Instead, she argued, people needed to be given the opportunity to "emancipate" themselves by "choosing to follow the new discoveries of nutrition."[60] As the committee later described, in a 1945 report, the central question guiding their work, "How can we change food habits?," made the individual the object of social change, rather than part of the process. They feared that this approach might lead toward "the type of authoritarianism in education and political practice which is incompatible with democracy." The report went so far as to suggest that this question "would have been a more appropriate question for the German Reich in 1936." The wrong kinds of methods, they worried, would result in the wrong kinds of citizens, fostering obedient, docile, and childlike attitudes about food, rather than the kind of responsible, self-reflective attitudes and behaviors that were appropriate for citizens in a democracy.[61]

In light of their concerns about the kinds of citizens lessons in eating right might shape, members of the Committee on Food Habits sought reform methods that were "consistent with the application of science in a democratic society."[62] Their approach was emblematic of what the historian William Graebner refers to as "democratic social engineering": "democratic" because it sought to modify beliefs and practices through a democratic process that included choice and participation, "social" because it often relied on group processes, and "engineering" because it made a conscious effort to control.[63] As the dominant system of authority in the United States throughout the twentieth century, democratic social engineering was particularly prevalent during the war years, as both concerns about authority and the need to maintain control were heightened. One of the landmark studies of democratic social engineering was in fact conducted by a member of the Committee on Food Habits, Kurt Lewin.[64] Lewin's study compared the effectiveness of the group-decision method, in which housewives participated in a discussion about feeding their families and were gently guided toward a predetermined conclusion by a facilitator, to that of lectures, which were considered more authoritarian. It found that guided group discussions produced even better results than did lectures, because women felt that they had independently come to conclusions about the kinds of changes they wanted to make in their families' diets. The method got results, but rather than instilling an ethos of rule following, it promoted the values of self-reflection and responsibility that were seen as hallmarks of democratic citizenship.[65]

The anxiety of hidden hunger combined with the ambition of the new RDAs to distribute the duty to eat right across the entire American population just in time for war. As a wartime propaganda campaign, the National Nutrition Program used the language of dietary reform to connect dietary ideals to wartime social ideals. Dietary self-improvement was like a pedagogy of good wartime citizenship, a way for people to both attain and express those qualities that were seen as most crucial on the home front, from courage and alertness to self-reflective responsibility. While addressing the eating habits of every single citizen was essential to the nutrition program's role as a morale campaign, it belied a more subtle emphasis on the eating habits of a subset of the population whose diets were considered most crucial to the war effort and, not surprisingly, most likely to be in need of reform.

Workers and Wives

The overalls and other elements of working-class dress on the family depicted on the Basic 7 food guide (see figure 3.1) would have made it clear to wartime Americans that eating right was a special duty for war workers. Despite its broad address, participatory structure, and democratic aims, the National Nutrition Program was not entirely reflective of the celebrated ideal of wartime pluralism. While it made eating right a duty for all Americans, the nutrition program also sought to contain the social dislocations of wartime, particularly those that threatened to disrupt hierarchies of class and gender. The war caused tremendous upheaval in the lives of most Americans and in the cultural mores and social structures that they had come to know and rely on. People's lives were dramatically altered as they responded to the simultaneous demands for soldiers on the battlefront and workers on the industrial front. Millions of families were uprooted as servicemen enlisted and jobseekers poured into cities looking for war work. Cities were strained by the influx of people looking for high-paying jobs, and tensions erupted as people vied for lucrative employment and scarce housing. African Americans increasingly found better, and better-paying, jobs. Old stereotypes were challenged by living and working conditions that brought new groups of people together, and the problems of race became the focus of intense national attention. The status of women also shifted perceptibly, as women took on war work and enjoyed new social and sexual freedoms on the home front.[66] Half of those polled in 1946 indicated that the war had changed their lives "a great deal," either positively or negatively. For many people, the experience of wartime, along with the changes it brought to daily life, led to a sense that stability was slipping away, leaving anxiety and chaos in its wake.[67] But even as mobilization produced such sources of anxiety and conflict, it required social cohesion and continuity.[68]

The nutrition program helped to secure cohesion and continuity of class and gender relations through programs aimed especially at workers and their wives. Insisting that the diets of workers posed a uniquely grave danger to the war effort, wartime reformers dedicated much of their effort to improving them, naturalizing class differences and gender roles through their assumptions, interventions, and conclusions. Concerns about the poor eating habits of workers grew out of an amalgam of nutritional and social concerns related to the mobilization and war effort. These concerns also played into the dynamic of middle-class self-making through the ongoing production of an "unhealthy other."[69] Risky, ignorant, and irresponsible eating habits among war workers were perceived as a major threat to the war effort because they jeopardized the nation's production and fighting capacity. But the perception of bad eating habits among workers also served the interest of social continuity by setting up an identity-affirming contrast.

The concern that war workers might not be physically fit for the massive job of defense ostensibly drove reformers to prioritize programs aimed at improving nutrition in industry. But anxieties about whether or not workers could be counted on to dedicate themselves adequately to the war effort informed these efforts as well. Concern about the diets of workers mirrored the concerns that domestic scientists had about the "character" of urban workers at the end of the nineteenth century. After a decade of economic hardship that saw massive increases in union membership, escalating militancy among workers, and federal protection of the workers' rights to organize and bargain collectively, the mobilization raised real concerns about the stability and cooperation of the labor force.[70] In 1941, with defense industries booming, more than two million workers went on strike—more than in any other year besides 1919 and 1937—and the Office of War Information warned, "If labor dissatisfaction is not reduced, workers will turn to more radical methods and more radical leaders."[71] The Nutrition in Industry program was launched that same year to respond to intertwined dietary and social concerns about whether workers could and would do their part.

Nutrition experts believed that war workers were predisposed toward poor dietary health and worried that in the context of the massive production demands of wartime they would be a weak link in the industrial machine on which victory depended. Depression-era research had convinced experts that while poor nutrition was a national problem, the diets of workers and the poor were in especially bad shape. Studies established, in essence, that workers were a woefully underfed and dangerously irresponsible "unhealthy other." In the early years of newer nutrition, researchers who wanted to know if people were getting enough nutrients had no proven methods to work with and often turned to expenditure as a way of measuring dietary adequacy. Because these studies assumed that the less people spent on food the less likely they were to be eating enough "protective foods," workers' diets were found to be especially lacking. A study conducted in forty-three industrial cities between 1934 and 1936, for example, found that among white workers' families only 11 to 21 percent had good diets, while 40 to 60 percent had poor diets.[72]

Not only did reformers believe that war workers were being drawn from a nutritionally compromised class of people, but they also worried that the Selective Service was leaving only the most poorly nourished of these men behind and, furthermore, that the conditions of war work would make matters even worse. Delegates at the National Nutrition Conference for Defense described workers entering defense industries, "many of whom have been rejected for military service," as "undoubtedly suffering from physical disabilities associated directly or indirectly with malnutrition such as underweight, general debility, defective teeth, and low-grade chronic infection." They went on to recommend "that steps be taken to condition nutritionally those classes of the population which are likely to become defense workers."[73] Later, the Committee on Nutrition in Industry, formed by the National Research Council, explained that workers were being drawn from the ranks of the poor and unemployed and taking jobs that required harder work, more effort, and in some cases longer hours and a longer work week than they were used to. Committee members worried that the poor health of these workers would only worsen, as many were going to be shifted from daytime to nighttime work and were likely to be employed in new plants located outside of existing communities, where normal housing, transportation, food, medical, and sanitation facilities were nonexistent.[74]

Concerns that wartime working conditions might exacerbate a propensity for bad eating habits among workers played out in relationship to the uncomfortable conviction that workers on the home front were just as critical to victory as soldiers on the battlefront. Wartime nutrition reformers insisted that the diets of defense-plant workers were absolutely critical to national security. Delegates at the National Nutrition Conference for Defense had established that "under modern conditions, those who forge the weapons of defense are just as important to our safety as those for whose use those weapons are intended."[75] The Committee on Nutrition in Industry confirmed the "strategic importance" of workers: "On their working efficiency depends to a considerable degree the hope of ultimate victory. . . . For the output of arms, munitions of every kind, and all the material needed in modern warfare, is dependent in the final analysis on the health and morale of these defense workers."[76] The sentiment was echoed repeatedly. An Office of War Information booklet called *Better Health: A Speedier Victory through Proper Nutrition* posed the hypothetical question "Why a National Nutrition Program?" and answered it: "Total war demands total strength. Our great civilian army of war workers must be kept strong and healthy. . . . Total strength demands proper nutrition."[77]

Convictions about the importance of workers' diets combined with existing beliefs about their inadequacy led to increased scrutiny and interventions that in the end only proved what reformers already knew—workers were not good eaters. Two programs, both launched in 1941 by Paul McNutt, administrator of the Defense Health and Welfare Services, simultaneously responded to and exacerbated concerns about the diets of war workers: the National Industrial Nutrition Program and the Advisory Service on Nutrition in Industry.[78] According to McNutt, the goal of the National Industrial Nutrition Program was to "reduce lost man hours on the production front," through programs that targeted three arenas: communities, industrial settings, and homes.[79] On the community front, the 48 state nutrition committees and 2,500 local nutrition committees already in operation were asked to prioritize the diets of workers in their jurisdictions.[80] Subcommittees on nutrition in industry dedicated themselves to reaching workers with nutritional information and messages about the importance of eating right as a wartime duty. They organized publicity programs through newspapers, magazines, plant publications, and radio broadcasts. They arranged lunch-box programs, neighborhood nutrition meetings for workers' wives and mothers, and meetings with restaurant and food-store owners. They oversaw the distribution of posters, flyers, and pledges of cooperation, and put together demonstrations of ideal factory canteens.[81] On the industrial front, the Advisory Service on Industrial Nutrition provided recommendations to both government-owned plants and private industries.[82] Its aims were to educate workers about what to eat and why, and to enable and encourage workers to obtain affordable, on-the-job meals that contained at least one-third of their daily dietary requirements, whether through a cafeteria, mobile or stationary canteens, or box lunches. Educational programs included rallies, talks, classes, demonstrations, consultations with dietitians, articles in plant publications, flyers, pamphlets, posters, and medical-history surveys designed to stimulate interest in nutrition.[83]

Efforts aimed at improving the eating habits of workers frequently reinforced the presumptive distinction between the healthy middle class and the irresponsible "unhealthy other" who simply could not be counted on to eat right. Reformers seeking to improve eating habits in industrial plants, for example, routinely reported on the bad habits they found there. They conducted nutrition studies in industrial plants to assess the needs for feeding and education programs, stimulate the interest of both workers and management in dietary problems, and obtain basic information for the education or in-plant feeding programs. But applying the extremely ambitious RDAs meant that they were likely to find poor eating habits wherever they looked. In a 1942 study researchers observed meals that workers chose from cafeteria lines in four Chicago-area war plants. They looked at 1,102 lunch trays in cafeterias where good food was provided for workers but found that only 8 percent of them chose adequate foods; 71 percent chose totally inadequate meals. These conclusions are not surprising, given that for a meal to be deemed adequate a worker had to select each of the following items from the available options: an eight-ounce glass of milk or two foods made from milk, each equivalent to one-half cup of milk; a three-quarter cup of green or yellow vegetables; one medium or two small potatoes; one serving of meat, cheese, fish, or eggs; two slices of whole-grain or enriched bread; one square of butter or fortified oleomargarine; and one of the following: 4.5 ounces tomato juice, 4.5 ounces grapefruit juice or one half grapefruit, one orange, 4.5–5 ounces raw cabbage or green pepper or a mixture of the two.[84] Calibrated to aim for "health-plus," the RDAs set up an impossible challenge for the workers whose diets became the central focus for wartime reformers. The inevitably disappointing findings among workers both legitimized the need for ongoing interventions and contributed to the sense that workers lacked the knowledge, will, and character to eat right.

After conducting studies to ascertain the effectiveness of the wartime nutrition program, reformers found that workers were not being adequately reached and concluded that they were somehow by nature disinclined to eat right. A 1942 study conducted by the USDA determined that most working-class wives had not been reached by nutrition education. Interviews suggested that working people "didn't think so much of that 'nutrition stuff'" and that in fact many of them thought nutrition was for people of "fancier" classes: "Among both working class men and their wives we found that nutrition was commonly associated with tea-room meals, attractive arrangement of food, and 'fancy' cooking. . . . Nutrition programs were 'cooking schools' attended by fashionable people, but not appropriate for a working man or his wife."[85] According to the study, working people thought that the nutrition programs were promoting diets that were impractical for working people, many working people did not attend public lectures on nutrition because of "hesitation about attending meetings with women of higher social status," and respondents found the meeting times and places inconvenient. The evidence suggested that the class connotations of nutrition-education programs were off-putting for working people. The researchers concluded that war workers —like the factory workers who had not seen the wisdom of the Indian pudding at the New England Kitchen—were disinclined to eat right because they were ignorant, stubborn, and complacent. The report stated that industrial workers "are, as a group, not anxious to be taught how to eat. Most of them are satisfied with the way they have always eaten. . . . They do not understand the concept of a balanced diet as a requirement for optimal vitality and resistance. . . . In their estimation a man who isn't sick and is eating enough to fill his stomach doesn't have to worry about food."[86] Describing workers as lacking "active interest," the report explained, "Although they think nutrition education is a good thing . . . they are not strongly impelled to do anything about it themselves."[87]

Like domestic scientists frustrated with their inability to change the habits of the "incorrigible" working class, wartime nutrition researchers stabilized the distinct identity of the healthy middle class by implying that workers were not eating right because they were irresponsible and indifferent. A report on the causes of malnutrition among war workers prepared by the Committee on Nutrition of Industrial Workers in 1945 cited inadequate income, physiological and metabolic disorders, unavailability of proper food, and "poor food habits." It went on to explain that poor food habits were caused by ignorance, improper selection or preparation, and indifference. Ignorance, the report argued, could be addressed through "mass activities to educate the people to select proper foods." People could learn to select whole or enriched grains and fresh or properly canned vegetables, and to prepare them in ways that maintained their vitamin content. But indifference seemed a more intractable problem. "Many workers have the money and enough knowledge to enable them to buy a good dietary and still fail to be well nourished because of their indifference," the report stated. "It is indifference that prompts a worker to rush through a breakfast of doughnuts and coffee when he knows that a leisurely meal of fruit, cereal, eggs and enriched bread is what he needs. . . . [It is] indifference that permits a housewife to serve the workers in her family an overcooked, drab dinner when she knows that overcooking impairs food values."[88]

The idea of poorly fed war workers established a moral hierarchy of class and character. Nutrition-education materials made it clear that eating right was closely related to good wartime citizenship, that the diets of defense workers were especially critical for defense, and that for workers, therefore, eating right was especially important to good citizenship. The social stakes of eating right were extremely high; the failure of workers to choose good diets due to ignorance or indifference was represented not just as a problem of individual health or productivity, but as a serious threat to the war effort. One striking piece of evidence makes this especially clear. *Eat Well to Work Well*, a booklet aimed at workers and their wives, included a section in which two facing pages compare good eaters to bad eaters (see figures 3.2 and 3.3). On one page is an image of a robust worker glowing with good health as he lunches on a sandwich, fruit, and milk, accompanied by text that reads, "Are You Helping Uncle Sam?" Underneath the image is a list of nutritional guidelines for good wartime citizenship, including, "Eat a hearty lunch every day to help keep you in top-notch physical condition, to make you feel like doing your job and 'playing ball' with your fellow workers." To help Uncle Sam, the worker is told, he should eat plenty of foods containing vitamin A (to keep vision clear), drink plenty of milk, choose "muscle-building" foods at lunch, drink plenty of water, get rest and fresh air, and, finally, "learn about food values. Regulate your diet and thus enjoy good health and live to a ripe

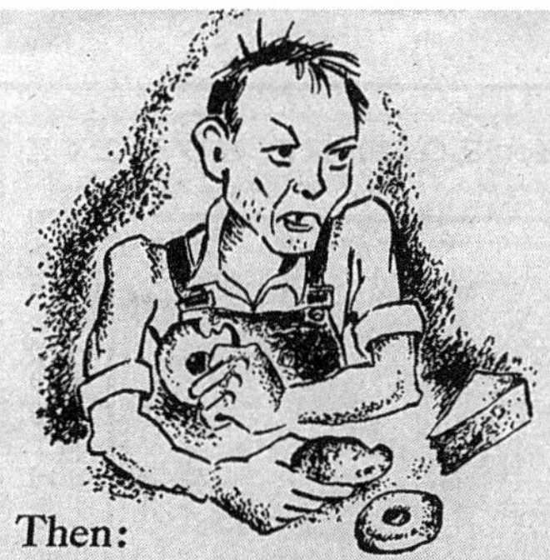

WORKER

Are You Helping Hitler?

Then:

Eat a poor lunch every day so that you will have many accidents, spoil much material, and keep your fellow-workers from getting their work done while you quarrel with them.

Eat only white bread—never whole-wheat or enriched. White bread has the fewest vitamins and will keep down your pep.

Don't eat eggs, liver, green vegetables, and yellow fruit; then the vitamin A in your eyes will be low. This will insure more accidents, because you see poorly. It may help you to smash your head or cut off your fingers.

Instead of thick sandwiches with good fillings, eat only a cake or a doughnut and some coffee for lunch. This may give you a headache by the end of the shift.

Don't eat oranges, tomatoes, cabbage, green peppers, or other fruits or vegetables in your lunch. Then you may get scurvy and your teeth may loosen. Dentists will then get too much of your pay check.

Let the other fellow drink your pint of milk each day. He will benefit from the calcium, protein, and vitamins in milk, and probably will do his work so well that the company will keep him busy after the war is over.

Don't eat sandwiches filled with peanut butter, liver, eggs, salmon, cheese, pork, beef, or chicken. These foods would keep your muscles in good condition, and you might feel as strong as a prize fighter and get more work done.

Don't drink much water; then the waste products in your body will accumulate in the blood and make you dopey. If you sweat a lot, don't eat extra salt—then you **really** will feel fatigued. This will keep you fighting with your boss so that he will not recommend you for promotion.

Don't wash your hands before eating; then you can get your peck of dirt. Swallow your food as fast as you can. You may have an iron stomach now but later on it may corrode and give you a goat's breath.

Don't learn anything about foods. If you do, you might choose a better diet, be able to forget your constipation, and quit fighting with your wife.

FIGURE 3.2 • High stakes for wartime eating right: nutritional treason. Clive McCay et al., "Eat Well to Work Well: The Lunch Box Should Carry a Hearty Meal," in *War Emergency Bulletin* 38; *Cornell Bulletin for Homemakers* 524 (1942).

WORKER

Are You Helping

Uncle Sam?

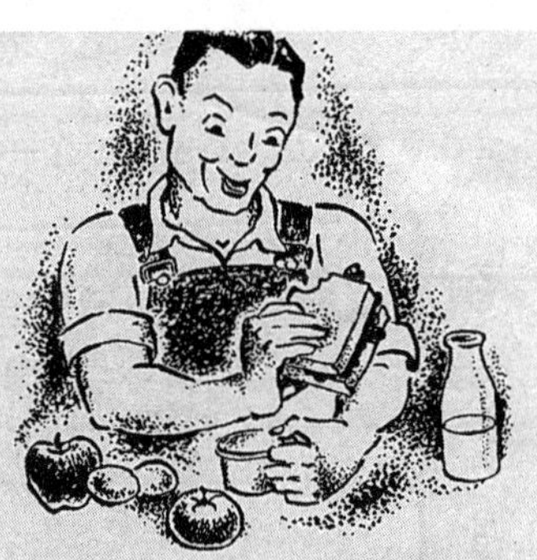

Then:

Eat a hearty lunch every day to help to keep you in top-notch physical condition, to make you feel like doing your job and "playing ball" with your fellow workers.

If possible, use whole-wheat bread. If you use white, be sure it is enriched with vitamins and iron. The slight extra money you pay is well worth the extra pep you get.

Keep your vision clear by eating plenty of green and yellow vegetables and fruits, salmon, and liver. These foods contain the vitamin A needed for good eyesight.

Make your lunch so hearty that it provides a large part of your day's need for vitamins, minerals, and proteins. The lunch period falls in the middle of your work day, and you need a good one to help you carry on. A good lunch is a good investment.

Include fruit in your lunch every day, such as an orange, apple, peach, or banana. Fresh or canned tomatoes and oranges help to protect you from scurvy.

Drink plenty of milk even if you feel that it is expensive. Remember it has many times the food value of any other drink.

Peanut butter, liver, eggs, salmon, cheese, pork, ham, beef, and chicken are muscle-building foods. Get one or two of these in your lunch every day. They will help to increase your capacity for work.

Plenty of water every day helps to flush waste products from the body. If you sweat a lot, drink extra water and eat extra salt to prevent fatigue.

Get plenty of rest and fresh air. Chew your food and eat slowly. Eat lunch with company you enjoy. Remember, no matter how good your lunch, it cannot give the best results if mixed with dirt and bacteria.

Learn about food values. Regulate your diet and thus enjoy good health and live to a ripe old age. You will have little trouble with constipation if your meals contain the vitamins in good meat, milk, and bread, as well as the roughage of vegetables and whole-grain cereals.

FIGURE 3.3 • High stakes for wartime eating right: nutritional patriotism. Clive McCay et al., "Eat Well to Work Well: The Lunch Box Should Carry a Hearty Meal," in *War Emergency Bulletin* 38; *Cornell Bulletin for Homemakers* 524 (1942).

old age." On the other page is a starkly different image: a skinny, haggard man, with sunken cheeks and a deranged expression, eating donuts and pie. Beside him, the text asks, "Are You Helping Hitler?" Underneath, a sarcastic set of nutritional instructions guide the bad wartime citizen: "Eat a poor lunch every day so that you will have many accidents, spoil much material, and keep your fellow-workers from getting their work done while you quarrel with them"; "Don't eat sandwiches filled with peanut butter, liver, eggs, salmon, cheese, pork, beef, or chicken. These foods would keep your muscles in good condition and you might feel strong as a prize fighter and get more work done"; and "Don't learn anything about foods. If you do, you might choose a better diet, be able to forget your constipation, and quit fighting with your wife." The pamphlet made it clear that the terms of good nutrition and good wartime citizenship were inseparable and that for workers the stakes involved in eating right, or not, were very high—there was certainly no worse form of wartime citizenship than the treason implied by the question, "Are you helping Hitler?"

While nutrition advice aimed at defense workers affirmed class distinctions, it also stabilized familiar gender roles and hierarchies. Despite the fact that the number of women who worked outside of the home rose by two million as military conscription created massive production demands on the home front, the nutrition program addressed women as essential because they were responsible for feeding workers, not because they were workers themselves.[89] The participation of women in war work—both industrial and civic—disrupted gender and familial norms, which were simultaneously strained by other changes associated with the demands of war. Families adjusted to geographic dislocations and changes in schedules, routines and provisions, and some sexual constraints on women gave way in the context of long male absences.[90] Though the Nutrition in Industry campaign contributed, if slightly, to wartime gender and familial alterations by moving some of the responsibility for feeding workers into factory canteens, its messages about food and health helped to contain these disruptions in traditional gender roles. It called on workers' wives not to "eat well to work well," but instead to become knowledgeable about the daily nutritional needs of their families, learn how to shop for nutritious foods despite changes in availability due to rationing and shortages, and learn how to prepare foods in order to conserve their vitamin content while making attractive and palatable dishes.

The nutrition discourse imagined good nutrition, and wartime citizenship, as something men achieved through the domestic service of wives and, therefore, situated the feeding of workers as a critical wartime duty for women. While soldiers in the army were being fed nutritionally sound rations based on the new RDAs, reformers worried that the war worker was at the mercy of his wife's uncertain nutritional knowledge and cooking ability. In November 1941 the *New York Times* reported that "Uncle Sam" was a "better feeder than housewives" and that, in fact, men in the army were better fed than 60 percent of the civilian population.[91] A Cornell radio brief reminded listeners, "He who does not eat the right food cannot work to his capacity." It went on to note, "About the man in the service we need not worry. . . . But you women who are both mess officer and company cook on the home front have a big responsibility resting in your kitchen right now."[92] The home was the third front in the battle for the health and vigor of workers. On launching the Industrial Nutrition Program, McNutt designated the home as one of three fronts in the battle for well-fed workers, the other two being communities and industrial settings. He called the home one of the program's most "vital points of attack" because it was where workers' lunches were packed. According to McNutt, "Over 8,000,000 lunches are packed for war workers every day. A big war job for American women is to see that these lunches contain the right food prepared to provide strength and health protection for American soldiers of production."[93]

The Committee on Food Habits articulated a theoretical justification for primarily addressing women in the nutrition campaign, although food reformers and advertisers alike had long since recognized women as their primary audience simply because they were typically responsible for shopping for food as well as preparing and serving it. The CFH member Kurt Lewin established the critical role of women in efforts to understand and influence eating habits in a paper based on a field study conducted in the spring and summer of 1942. The paper, "Forces behind Food Habits and Methods of Change," argued that understanding "why people eat what they eat" must start with understanding "how food comes to the table and why," because once food appears on the table, most of it gets eaten, regardless of quality. "Channel theory" detailed the various ways that food came to the table and established that in order to influence food habits social scientists needed to understand the psychology of the "gatekeeper" who controlled those channels. "In all our groups," Lewin explained, referring to the five economic and cultural groups studied, "the wife definitely controls all the channels except that of gardening and even there the husband rarely controls this channel alone." Because the wife was understood to be the keeper of the channels through which food arrived at the table, where it was inevitably eaten, it was her behavior that needed to be changed in order to influence the eating habits of the nation.[94]

Interviews conducted as part of a USDA study to assess the impact of the nutrition program suggested that men and women understood that providing good nutrition for workers was the duty of wives. One man explained that it was not his job to know what a person needed to eat: "That's something I hardly pay attention to. I just go to the table and take what I want. . . . They have programs on the radio about food but I never pay attention. I feel that's a woman's place."[95] In another conversation the interviewer asked a couple if there were any foods they ate because they were supposed to be good for you. While the husband replied that there were not, that he could "eat anything," the wife said, "I do the planning and I sure do it. I don't understand how he can say that. I have my vitamin charts and pamphlets that I watch and see that he gets the proper food."[96]

The Industrial Nutrition Program managed gender disruptions by suggesting that women's domestic service was an important component of dietary health for workers and, by extension, that victory depended on the maintenance of such gender hierarchy. In some cases women were called on to feed themselves and their families well, but the duty to serve husbands and children good food was usually emphasized. The conflation of domestic service to men and children with patriotic service to the nation was especially clear in a pledge sheet distributed by the New York Federation of Home Bureaus. The pledge states, "I am a Kitchen Kommando—a homemaker in the SERVICE OF MY COUNTRY. My goal is to make my family strong by feeding my family well. As a Kitchen Kommando I will serve my family simple, nutritious meals, using the 'daily food guide' to help me plan" (see figure 3.4). The pledge also includes promises to avoid wasting and hoarding and to recruit at least one other homemaker as a Kitchen Kommando within six weeks.[97] The sheet is illustrated with a picture of a squadron of Kitchen Kommandos waving American flags, holding wooden spoons instead of rifles, and wearing uniforms of aprons with front pockets bearing the initials "KK."

A nutrition poster issued in 1944 also suggested that female service and traditional gender roles were critical to good nutrition (see figure 3.5). The poster comprises three sections that correspond to the following text: "For

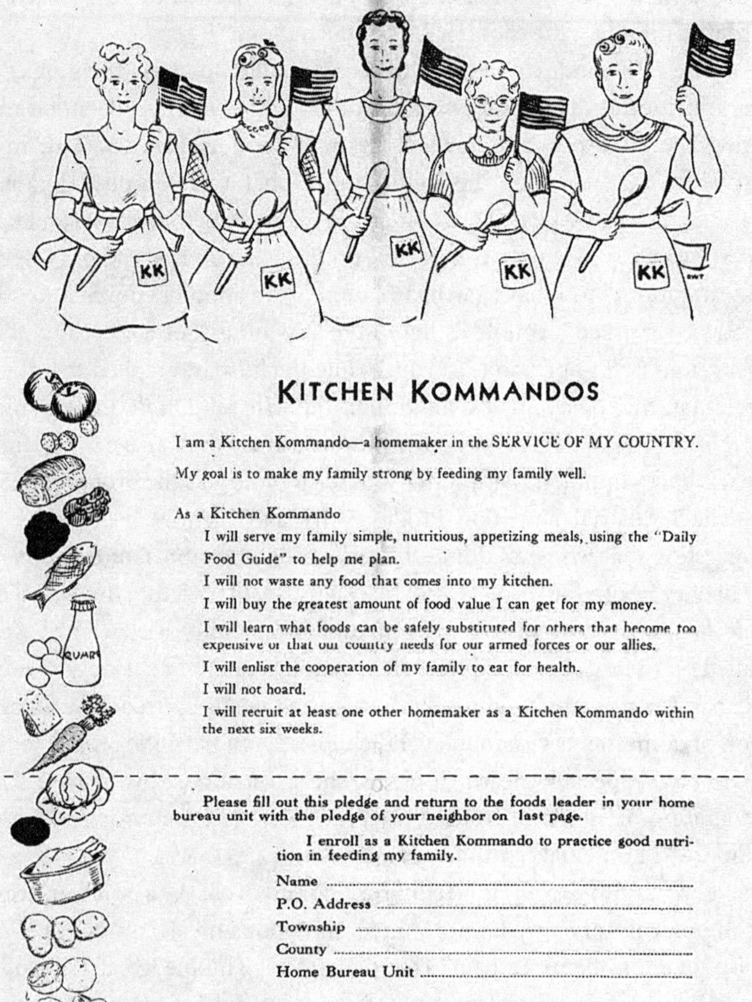
KITCHEN KOMMANDOS

I am a Kitchen Kommando—a homemaker in the SERVICE OF MY COUNTRY.

My goal is to make my family strong by feeding my family well.

As a Kitchen Kommando

I will serve my family simple, nutritious, appetizing meals, using the "Daily Food Guide" to help me plan.

I will not waste any food that comes into my kitchen.

I will buy the greatest amount of food value I can get for my money.

I will learn what foods can be safely substituted for others that become too expensive or that our country needs for our armed forces or our allies.

I will enlist the cooperation of my family to eat for health.

I will not hoard.

I will recruit at least one other homemaker as a Kitchen Kommando within the next six weeks.

Please fill out this pledge and return to the foods leader in your home bureau unit with the pledge of your neighbor on last page.

I enroll as a Kitchen Kommando to practice good nutrition in feeding my family.

Name ....

P.O. Address ....

Township ....

County ....

Home Bureau Unit ....

Sponsored by the New York State Federation of Home Bureaus.

FIGURE 3.4 • Kitchen Kommandos: a wartime division of nutritional citizenship. New York State College of Home Economics records, #23–2–749. Division of Rare and Manuscript Collections, Cornell University Library.

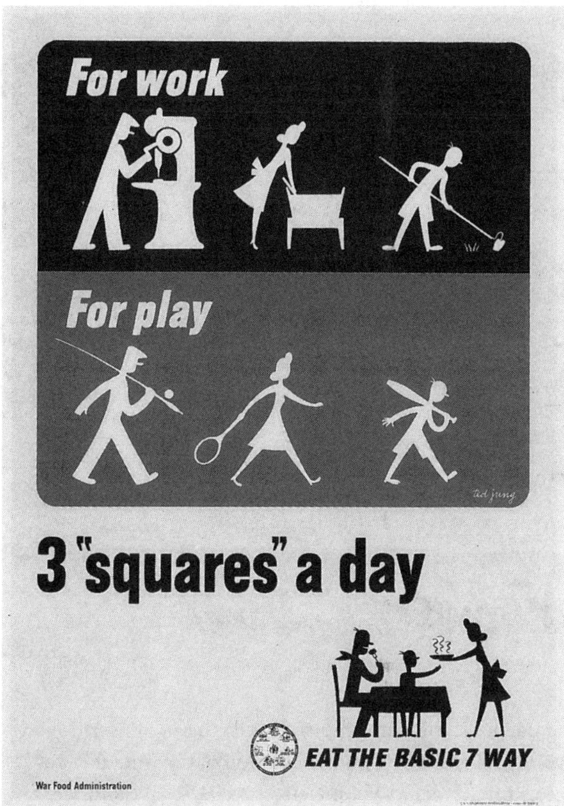

FIGURE 3.5 • Female service as part of eating "the Basic 7 way." University of North Texas Digital Library.

work . . . For play . . . 3 'squares' a day." The first two sections show a working-class mother, father, and son engaged in clearly gendered activities. In the "For work," section, for example, a man works an industrial machine, a woman labors over a washtub, and a boy hoes a garden. In the final section, under the heading "3 'squares' a day," the woman provides a meal for her husband and her son. The man and boy are both sitting at a table, and the man is bringing a forkful of food to his mouth while the boy reaches toward a steaming plate being offered to him by his mother. The woman stands next to the table wearing an apron and serving her family, but there appears to be no place for her at the table.[98]

The grand social ambitions of the wartime food program, the conflation of wartime dietary and social ideals, the special concern about workers' diets and the expectation of female domestic service were all beautifully illustrated in a single image in a 1941 issue of the USDA *Consumer's Guide*. Titled "Mrs. America Volunteers" the issue focused on preparing

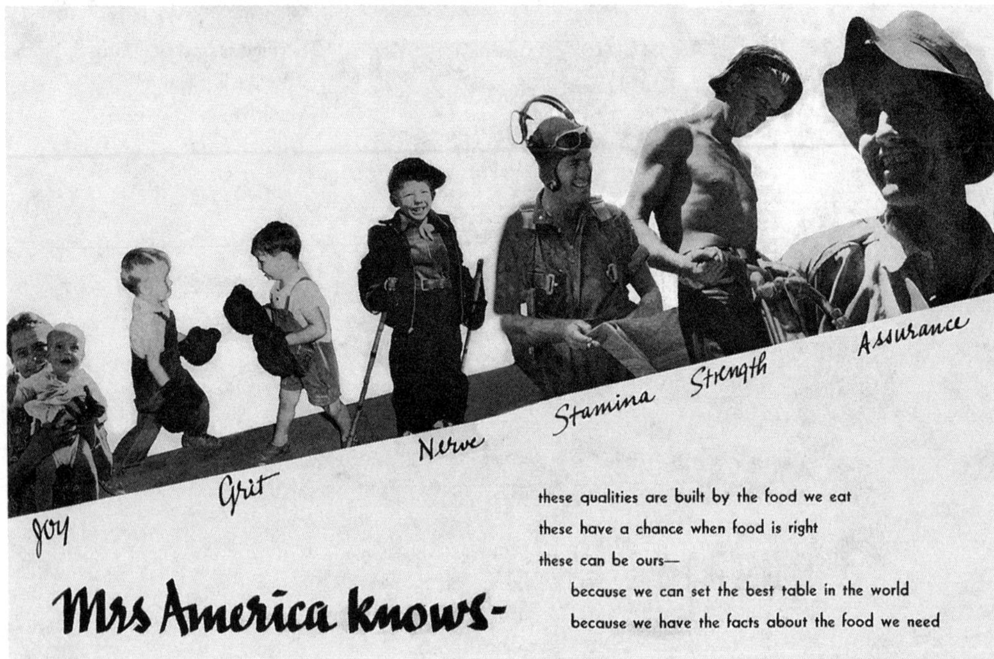

FIGURE 3.6 • Celebrating the potential, both empirical and ethical, of nutrition in the hands of American women. Consumer Counsel Division of the United States Department of Agriculture, "Mrs. America Volunteers," special issue, *Consumer's Guide* 7, no. 20 (October 15, 1941).

women for the wartime work of feeding their families. It taught "Mrs. America" to buy with care, plan with care, and prepare with care, explaining, "There's victory in victuals!" The issue opened with a two-page spread that dramatized many of the arguments I have made about the social role of wartime dietary reform (see figure 3.6). Across the pages are a series of photos depicting the life development of a male: an infant in his mother's arms, boxing toddlers, a boy in skiing clothes, a young man in aviation gear, a bare-chested man working a jackhammer, and a fully mature man. Beneath each image is a word that captures one of the qualities of good wartime citizenship that women were being called on to foster through good food: joy, grit, nerve, stamina, strength, assurance. The body of the text celebrates the awesome potential, both empirical and ethical, of nutritional knowledge in the hands of American women: "Mrs. America knows: these qualities are built by the foods we eat. These have a chance when food is right. These can be ours—because we can set the best table in the world. Because we have the facts about the food we need."[99]

THE WAR MARKED a turning point in American nutritional discourse; the discovery of vitamins and "hidden hunger" dovetailed with the exigencies of war to emphasize the problem of eating right and expand the purview of dietary reformers to the entire population. With its demands for both physical fortitude and social cohesion, the context of war put new pressures on both the empirical and the ethical aspects of nutrition, producing a discourse that seamlessly integrated new facts about the importance of vitamins with home-front ideals of good citizenship.

In an empirical sense, today's ideas about what to eat are a world away from wartime ideals. The Basic 7 food guide does not mention that some foods are better than others; there are no foods to avoid, no dangers posed by too much of certain nutrients or additives, and there is an entire food group dedicated to butter! (And margarine, which served as its substitute for practical, not medical reasons.)[100] But what it means to be fat or to shop at a farmers market today emerges as much from the foundation of scientific morality laid by domestic scientists and the expansions in the scope and significance of dietary reform that took place during the war years as it does from contemporary nutritional and social concerns. A series of realignments in the postwar years ushered in a new set of nutritional guidelines that favored some foods and demonized others (like butter), shifted the focus from nutritional deficiency to excess, and even paved the way for questions about the dominance of nutritional thinking in defining "good food." Alongside these changes were growing concerns about the relationship between "lifestyle" and health and related transformations in the meaning of good citizenship. Two very different dietary reforms took shape in this context: the alternative food movement and the antiobesity movement. Both of them not only built on but also radically expanded the social role and cultural meaning of eating right they inherited from the dietary-reform movements of the first half of the twentieth century.

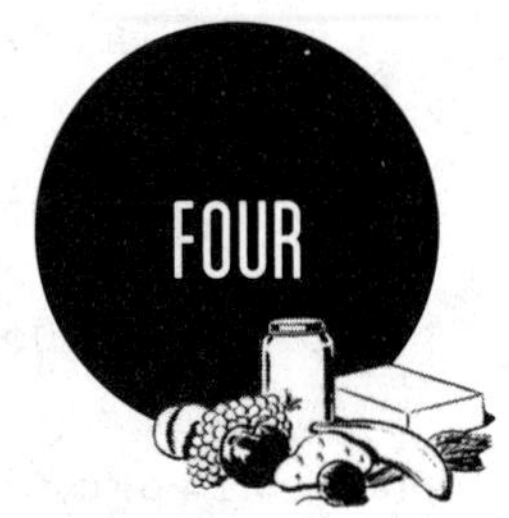

FROM MICROSCOPES TO "MACROSCOPES"

By 1980, when the Columbia professor of nutrition and education Joan Dye Gussow was invited to give the fourth presentation in the annual Ellen Swallow Richards Lecture Series, sponsored by the Institute of Nutrition at the University of North Carolina, she was already well known for advancing the idea that "good food" was not simply a matter of nutrients.[1] But looking back on Ellen Richards's life and work gave her an occasion to articulate the distinctions between the approach to dietary health that Richards had ushered in and the radical rethinking of eating right that was taking shape. Gussow explained that in preparation for her talk she had done a little background research on Ellen Richards and discovered that "the mother of home economics" was responsible for leading women toward the "scientification of food," whereby food was slowly but surely reduced to the value of its nutrients. For Gussow, the focus on nutrients that Richards had championed no longer seemed an adequate means of understanding dietary health or defining a good diet. She warned that scientists had for too long focused on "microscopic pieces; looking at the isolated effects of the isolated behaviors on isolated food substances in isolated biological systems." Instead, she argued, "I believe it is time now for some of us . . . to take up our macroscopes instead of our microscopes." According to Gussow, this broader lens would shift attention from the connections between "nutrients and cells" to the connections between food and a host of other issues. Dietary health would no longer be seen as a strictly nutritional calculus, but would take into account the connections between "farmers and producers; between food policies and environmental policies; between toxic wastes and the opportunity to produce safe, affordable food[;] . . . between the cost of energy and the cost of food." With these connections in mind, Gussow argued, nutritionists should engage in a major rethinking of the food system, considering alternatives to the industrial food system, exploring the possibility of a localized food supply, and planning for the long-term future of affordable and nutritious food.[2]

Nutrition remained an important lens for thinking about dietary health, but by the end of the twentieth century a dietary-reform movement that drew on the intellectual roots laid by Gussow and others of her era had emerged to champion a macroscopic view of good food. This "movement" in reality comprised many different movements that shared a critical view of the industrial food system, skepticism about the narrow nutritional definition of a good diet, and an understanding of dietary health as inseparable from other forms of well-being (environmental, social, economic). Collectively referred to as the "alternative food movement," these efforts promoted ecologically sound production methods, conscientious consumption, and local economies by supporting various means of connecting small-scale producers of organically grown, local, fresh, and artisan-produced foods with consumers over the shortest distance possible. Projects were often oriented around supporting the sites where these connections occurred, such as farmers markets and community-supported agriculture, and cultivating a receptive public through advocacy, education, and marketing.[3] I focus here on what might reasonably be called the tip of this iceberg, that is, the most mainstream and iconic articulations of an ethos of eating right that focused on the links between individual bodies, biological systems, and social and economic well-being. My approach is reductive, and I necessarily overlook many complexities in a strategic attempt to extract, distill, and analyze an important cultural shift in the definition of a good diet, in the meaning of eating right, and in the scope and purview of dietary reform.[4]

In the context of alternative food, the emphasis of dietary advice shifted from the empirical to the ethical, the epistemology of eating right shifted from nutrition to ecology, and the reference point of a good diet shifted from physiology to the food system. In addition to challenging nearly a century of nutritional thinking as the guiding principle of dietary advice by embracing a primarily ethical approach to eating right, alternative food also incorporated, rather than rejected, pleasure. Since the ethos of alternative food situated dietary health at the center of a complex social, economic, and environmental matrix, a good diet was no longer defined by its ability to fuel the body efficiently, as it had been the Progressive Era, or to promote optimum health, as it had been in during the Second World War. Instead, eating right was understood to emerge from a nexus of knowledge about where food came from, responsible choices based on that knowledge, and pleasure that both guided and derived from those choices. But the redefinition of eating right around the knowledge-pleasure-responsibility nexus was less a departure from the narrative of dietary reform that began with domestic science and continued in the National Nutrition Program than it appeared to be. Despite its rejection of nutritional norms, casting off of rules, emphasis on ethics and celebration of pleasure, this redefinition of eating right did not diminish the empirical role played by dietary advice and it played a role in extending, once again the purview and significance of dietary norms in American life. The self-making aspects of eating right were central to alternative-food discourse, which celebrated eating as an ethical act and promoted the links between eating right and responsible citizenship. Less obvious were connections between lessons in eating right and the values of neoliberalism, as well as the role that alternative dietary ideals played in naturalizing class through a moral hierarchy of dietary health.

Redefining a Good Diet: Knowledge, Responsibility, and Pleasure

The late-twentieth-century redefinition of dietary health through a "macroscopic" lens drew on deep ideological roots. Currents of social activism related to food purity and agriculture, dating back to the pure-food movements of the Progressive Era and the Depression years respectively, converged in alternative food. Environmentalism also played a major role in shaping the movement's concerns and convictions.[5] The ecologically oriented, oppositional politics of alternative food were also very much shaped by the social movement Warren Belasco calls "the countercuisine," a corollary to the counterculture that focused on food as a means of social action and personal expression. As Belasco explains, environmentalism and ecology emerged quite suddenly "as the left's primary vehicle for outrage and hope" between 1969 and 1970, as civil rights, the antiwar movement, and revolutionary socialism stagnated, fragmented, or otherwise lost widespread appeal. Ecology transcended the divisiveness of the other movements and brought food to the center of the era's idealism. It gave people a way to respond to a sense of widespread social disorder and environmental crisis, offering tangible steps that people could act on immediately, such as changing their eating habits. Dietary change was an appealing, accessible, and powerful way radicals could state their opposition to mainstream, industrial values and remake their world in more ecological terms. The countercuisine generated a series of oppositions—such as "natural" vs. "plastic," "brown" vs. "white," "slow foods" vs. "fast food"—through which radicals constructed their identity in contrast to mainstream cuisine and values.[6]

Against this backdrop, a handful of influential writers and thinkers began to articulate the holistic reconceptualization of eating right that would eventually animate alternative food. They redefined health as transcending the biomedical status of individual bodies and dietary health as inextricably related to ecological and social well-being. Wendell Berry, a writer who was born on a Kentucky farm and began tending his own homestead in 1965, started publishing essays about agriculture around 1970. His eloquent writing helped establish the idea that food—and therefore dietary health—was at the center of an elaborate agricultural and social matrix. He revitalized the work of Sir Albert Howard, who would become known as the founder of modern organic agriculture, advocating for replacing the fragmented approach of scientific agriculture with a "synthetic approach" that looks at "the wheel of life as one great subject and not as if it were a patchwork of unrelated things." Citing Howard, Berry famously argued we should understand "the whole problem of health in soil, plant, animal and man as one great subject."[7] From this perspective, the quality of food was clearly not determined by nutrition alone. It was "indistinguishable from *health*—bodily health, coming from good food, but also economic, political, cultural, and spiritual health."[8] In *Diet For a Small Planet*, published in 1971, Frances Moore Lappé also offered a view of dietary health that transcended the question of individual bodies, connecting the dinner table of average Americans to issues of global food supply. The book, which eventually sold close to two million copies, redefined good food in terms of the impact of its production on the well-being of the earth and argued for a vegetarian diet as the least wasteful of natural resources.[9] In 1978 Gussow published her classic *The Feeding Web: Issues in Nutritional Ecology*, which highlighted the environmental dangers of the global food system. Later, in a 1982 essay, Gussow bluntly conveyed the urgency of redefining "good food" beyond the traditional constraints of nutritional thinking: "Either someone thinks about the system as a whole . . . or we simply go on pretending nutrition has only to do with what happens after food leaves the throat, ignoring the aberrations of a system so vulnerable to human error that it may one day soon leave us short of wholesome food to put in our mouths."[10]

The ecological understanding of good food and expansive view of health developed by these pioneering thinkers was, for a number of reasons, reinvigorated at the end of the century. Ecological ideals—along with several other factors, including profit incentives—had driven a growing interest in the consumption and production of organically produced foods throughout the 1980s and 1990s.[11] But by the start of the new century angst about what to eat was on the rise and the desire to create alternatives to the industrial food system was far exceeding organics (which, to the dismay of many of its early proponents, had itself been industrialized).[12] Concerns about the safety of industrial food, heightened by a series of high-profile scares in the late 1980s, were enflamed in 2001 by the publication of Eric Schlosser's *Fast Food Nation*, with its captivating and disgusting expose of the fast food industry.[13] In 2002 Marion Nestle's *Food Politics* undermined confidence in dietary recommendations by exposing the politics behind the federal nutritional guidelines.[14] Meanwhile, legislative changes throughout the 1990s had increased health claims exponentially, leading to a proliferation of new foods, new terms, and new anxieties for consumers.[15] As concerns about the safety and quality of food intensified, alarm about rising rates of overweight and obesity drew even more unflattering attention to the American diet and the industrial food system behind it. Concerns about the safety and sustainability of the industrial system of food production were amplified in the context of growing scientific, political, and cultural attention to global warming and other disturbing signs that ongoing industrial exploitation of the environment was simply not going to be possible. Nervous about industrial food and losing confidence in mainstream dietary advice, American food consumers (of a certain class) rediscovered the ideas about good food that had once propelled the countercuisine. By the beginning of the twenty-first century, a new definition of dietary health, oriented around the concept of connection and a critique of industrialization, was manifesting in a myriad of independent but ideologically sympathetic publications, organizations, and projects, and beginning to take the shape of a dietary-reform movement.

Responding to the growing distrust of the industrial food system, high-profile figures such as Alice Waters and Michael Pollan generated and popularized new definitions of "good food." Waters developed both a cuisine and an ethos of eating right that emphasized the links between good food and agricultural practices guided by the kinds of connections Berry's writing illuminated. Her ideas emerged in part from her experience as an exchange student in France, where she experienced a different relationship to eating and began to think about the connections between a culture's values and its eating habits. She was moved by the freshness of the food, its simple preparation, and the time people took out of their days to enjoy meals with friends and family. Back in Berkeley, where Waters was a student immersed in the Free Speech movement, she decided to open a small café and restaurant to feed her community of Berkeley bohemians.[16]

Chez Panisse opened in 1971, and Waters's ethos of eating right evolved in response to the practical constraints she and the other cooks faced as they tried to reproduce French home cooking. Unable to find the quality of produce they felt they needed, they blamed economies of scale for prioritizing profit over flavor and identified the distance between producers and consumers—both literal and figurative—as a major social and dietary problem. Working outside of the normal channels, the staff strove to eliminate the distance, delays, and anonymity of the industrial food system by developing what they would call a "hunter gatherer culture," where employees "foraged" for the finest, freshest local delicacies.[17] Soon Chez Panisse staff recognized that the best ingredients were coming from environmentally responsible growers. They developed a network of suppliers who were able to meet their demands for fresh, tasty ingredients and established a set of principles for suppliers that included not only flavor and freshness but also farming practices. They began to consciously build what Waters described as not merely a supply network, but a "community of people who share our goals of providing fresh, perfectly grown foods while promoting sustainable agriculture that takes care of the earth."[18] Throughout the 1970s and 1980s, Waters used the restaurant's fixed menu and the many cookbooks she published to teach diners about the connections between good food and good farming practices.[19] By the mid-1990s, she was working to bring the new concept of a good diet to the American public through activism and advocacy.

A journalist who began writing about food in the early 2000s, Michael Pollan popularized the concept of eating as an engagement with the natural world and brought the notion that nutrition was an inadequate measure of good food to the American public. In *The Omnivore's Dilemma*, published in 2006, Pollan gave readers an intimate look at three different food chains—industrial, organic or alternative, and hunter-gatherer—and suggested that eaters had a choice about what kind of world to endorse through the meals they chose. The book advocated an ecological view of good food and cast suspicion on the "health" of the industrial food system.[20] Two years later, in *In Defense of Food*, Pollan connected the problems of industrial food to narrow nutritional thinking about dietary health, critiquing what he referred to as the "Nutritional Industrial Complex." Echoing Gussow and Berry, Pollan argued that a reductive, fragmented view of food quality and dietary health led to the acceptance of industrially produced "food-like substances" that technically met nutritional requirements but were entirely unhealthy through the broader view of dietary health. Drawing on the work of the Australian critic Gyorgy Scrinis, Pollan described an "ideology of nutritionism" that had naturalized a view of food as a composite of nutrients and the notion that biomedical health was the primary aim of eating. "Nutritionism," he argued, eclipsed other modes of assessing the value of food—such as ecology, tradition, culture, and history—to our grave peril.[21]

As Waters, Pollan, and others imagined alternatives to the industrial food system and to nutritionism's narrow view of the relationship between food and health, they also redefined the relationship between pleasure and eating right. Domestic scientists dismissed pleasure as a danger to right eating, only occasionally ceding that the appeal of food to the senses might play a role in the digestive process. For Second World War–era reformers, an ethos of wartime sacrifice made pleasure more or less irrelevant. And within antiobesity discourse, the denial of pleasure was seen as a key to dietary health. Alternative food reformers, however, believed that knowledge about food origins would provide a foundation both for choosing foods responsibly and for delighting in the experience of eating good food. The deliciousness of responsibly sourced foods might also lead to curiosity about food origins, which could (and should) result in responsible choices, and thus in more pleasure. The idea that sensual pleasure was key to eating right promised a kind of liberation from the kitchen-as-laboratory ideal that domestic scientists cherished and from the rule-bound rationality of science-based dietary norms. But it meant that for the first time in the history of modern dietary reform, pleasure was to be directed rather than denied. With pleasure essential to eating right, the purview of dietary reform expanded to reach deep within the subjectivity of individual eaters.

The mandate to find rather than deny pleasure in eating right was first articulated by Wendell Berry in his widely anthologized essay "The Pleasure of Eating" (1989), which both Pollan and Waters would later cite, celebrate, and build on.[22] In the essay Berry famously argued that eating was "an agricultural act" and explained that eating right thus required deliberate, informed, and responsible choices having to do not simply with nutrition, but with the entire social and physical matrix in which food was located. Understanding where food came from and being as directly involved in its production as possible was, therefore, not only a duty but also a source of true pleasure. Distinct from "the pleasure of the gourmet," this pleasure of eating right was an "extensive pleasure" that might evoke the beauty of the garden, gratitude for the source of the food, or the comfort of knowing of the good health of the plot or pasture from which the food was produced. For Berry, the pleasure of eating was a fundamental aspect of dietary health—what he referred to as perhaps "the best available standard of our health"—because it signified and cemented the connection between the eater, the food being eaten, and its origins. Not just any pleasure, but pleasure connected to knowledge about where food came from, was essential to eating ethically. As Berry so eloquently argued, "Eating with the fullest pleasure—pleasure, that is, that does not depend on ignorance—is perhaps the profoundest enactment of our connection with the world."[23]

Building on this fundamental understanding of pleasure as an accessory to ethical eating, Alice Waters described her job as a restaurateur as exposing people to the pleasure of good food in order to lead them toward responsible choices about what to eat. In explaining the importance of pleasure in eating right, she often used the story of her first taste of *fraises des bois* (wild strawberries, literally "strawberries of the woods") as an exchange student in France: "My eyes fluttered shut and I did not know what to say. It had never occurred to me that strawberries originally came from the woods nor that I was deeply connected with nature." Waters described this experience as having presented her, all at once, "a glimmer of understanding of the truth that Wendell Berry would express so well years later."[24] Building on her conviction that eating with pleasure —"pleasure, that is, that does not depend on ignorance"—was essential to eating right, Waters used Chez Panisse to "awaken" people's senses and introduce them to responsible eating by providing experiences like the one she had tasting those first fraises des bois in France. The restaurant's unusual structure—a single, unique meal offered each night at a fixed price—allowed Waters to use her cooking to methodically influence the eating habits of its patrons, and she also preached the importance of pleasure and sensuality in her cookbooks, essays, and interviews.[25] For Waters, like Berry, the pleasure of good food was not frivolous. Waking people up to the pleasure of food was a means of illuminating the matrix of connections within which food was embedded and thus of teaching them to make responsible choices about what to eat.

This concept of eating right foregrounded pleasure and ethics; the quantitative, rule-bound empiricism of nutrition-driven dietary ideals seemed nowhere to be found. The new concept of eating right did not, however, vanquish empiricism. Rather, it reversed the relationship more common to the modern dietary-reform movement. Instead of obscuring the ethical in the empirical, promoting quantitative measures that expressed moral values, it obscured the empirical in the ethical. There were no numerical charts comparing cost to nutritional value (like Atwater's) or precise daily allowances for nutrients (as with the war-era RDAs), but there were dietary norms subtly embedded within the idea of moral pleasure. The purpose of pleasure was ethical eating, not hedonism; indeed, some pleasures were considered antithetical to eating right.

However delectable a fast-food burger and fries may have been to some, proponents of alternative food considered the pleasures of cheap, fast, processed food to be the unfortunate outcome of the industrial food system's relentless manipulation of people's desires through deceptively cheap, flavor-engineered foods. Waters, for example, described the senses as a compass that, if given the chance, would inevitably steer people away from the deluded, pathetic "pleasures" of industrial food and back to the real pleasures of simple, wholesome cuisine. The bottom line of change, she remarked, was simply to "open [people's] senses so that they can make decisions. I have an underlying faith that once having had good food put before them, they'll choose the good."[26] Pollan also argued that pleasure derived from food knowledge was not only essential to eating right, but also a more true form of pleasure than that which came from ignorant consumption of industrial food: "To eat with a fuller consciousness of all that is at stake might sound like a burden, but in practice few things in life can accord quite as much satisfaction. By comparison, the pleasures of eating industrially, which is to say eating in ignorance, are fleeting."[27]

The subtle empiricism of eating with great pleasure surfaced in the new rules that Pollan proposed to replace nutritionism. *In Defense of Food* made famous his dictum "Eat food. Mostly plants. Not too much," which provided the empirical guidelines through which the ethical work of eating right was to take place. As Pollan explained, his "rules of thumb" were designed to provide an ecological and cultural approach to "the food problem."[28] They expanded on the general idea that instead of worrying about nutrients, people should avoid processed foods, focus on a broader concept of health, and revert to the more labor intensive but satisfying eating habits of the past. Pleasure, as Pollan explained, was central. The rules were "conducive not only to better health but also to greater pleasure in eating, two goals that turn out to be mutually reinforcing."[29] His *Food Rules: An Eater's Manifesto* (2009) and an expanded illustrated version published a few years later provided even more rules along these same lines, further capitalizing on the growing appeal of rules for eating right that both foregrounded and linked pleasure and ethics.[30]

While the idea of eating for pleasure may have seemed to liberate people from the binding self-denial of scientific nutrition, this approach to eating right replaced the quantifiable norms of other reform movements with qualitative ones that were no less normative. But because these dietary ideals included a mandate to enjoy a good diet, the internal landscape of preference, taste, and pleasure now fell under the purview of dietary reform. Being a good eater within this new set of ideals required that individuals reform not only their behaviors, but also their desires. With these inroads into the subjectivities of individual eaters, the movement marked out new terrain in the scope of dietary reform.

This expansion in the scope of dietary reform was amplified by an overall increase in the social and moral valence of eating habits that had taken place since the end of the Second World War. These changes reoriented health promotion around individual behaviors and lifestyle choices, bringing new levels of scrutiny to all health-related practices, but especially to eating habits. After World War II, the focus of the health community shifted away from contagious diseases and a primarily biomedical conception of health, to chronic diseases (cancer, diabetes, cardiovascular disease) and an approach to health that also encompassed social and environmental factors. Many called this a "second public-health revolution" because it restored the environmental focus of the first public-health revolution, which occurred in response to the problems of industrialization at the beginning of the twentieth century and informed the work of domestic scientists.

The renewed emphasis on environmental conditions that were believed to promote and inhibit health also entailed a persistent focus on individual behaviors within those environments. By the late 1960s, concerns about chronic disease, smoking, environmental degradation, and the safety of the food supply had brought health to the center of American culture and politics. Increasing anxiety about these threats to health led to interest in both government regulation of industry and the management of individual health risks through behavioral change, but in the end the message of personal responsibility prevailed.[31] Anticorporate calls for regulation of health hazards generated political controversies and amplified the public's sensitivity to lifestyle dangers. While corporations resisted the push for legislation, they were eager to capitalize on the new discourse of personal responsibility for health. This led to the emergence of what Robert Crawford calls the "new health consciousness," an "ideological formation that defined problems of health and their solutions principally, although not exclusively, as matters within the boundaries of personal control."[32] At the same time, the cultural condition known as "healthism" was coming into being, as the range of behaviors considered health-related expanded and health became increasingly culturally and socially salient. The prevention of illness became a pervasive standard against which an expanding number of behaviors and phenomenon were judged. This broadening of the understanding of health in the late twentieth century redefined everything from seatbelt and helmet use to smoking and advertisements for alcohol as health-related practices and brought them under the purview of public-health legislation and reform. As Crawford explains, both the pursuit of health and the state of being "healthy" became increasingly important to people's everyday lives, their self-definition, and their moral assessment of themselves and others.[33]

Alongside the emergence of healthism, changes in the prevailing nutritional paradigm positioned eating right as a particularly important health practice.[34] Following World War II the nutrition community realized that research into vitamin deficiency had been exhausted, and in the late 1960s nutritionists began to regroup around the relationship between diet and illness such as cardiovascular disease, cancer, and diabetes. The vitamin-oriented nutritional thinking that had guided wartime reformers was supplanted by a new paradigm that Belasco calls "negative nutrition." Eating too few vitamin-rich "protective" foods had been deemed dangerous because it could lead to both acute and chronic forms of malnutrition, but it turned out that eating *too much* of certain foods could also be bad for dietary health. In 1969 the White House Conference on Food, Nutrition and Health included some discussion of deficiency diseases, but emphasized and brought new levels of public attention to the dietary determinants of what participants called "the health problems of adults in an affluent society—the degenerative diseases of middle age."[35] Recommendations to eat less of foods high in fat, sugar, cholesterol, and salt emerged from the conference. In 1973 national attention was again brought to the relationship between diet and disease, by a series of hearings on how diet affected obesity, diabetes, and heart disease. Yet another series of hearings in which witnesses described the health risks involved in eating too much of the wrong kinds of food was held in 1976. The name of the hearings distilled the concerns of the emerging nutritional paradigm: "Diet Related to Killer Diseases." Eating right, increasingly defined by the avoidance of potentially harmful foods, gained national attention as a primary means through which individuals could practice and pursue health. As health practices in general were elevated to a new level of social significance, dietary behavior was increasingly considered central to both the biomedical achievement of health and the status of being "healthy."

It was against this backdrop that the alternative food movement capitalized on the notions, quickly becoming common sense, that health came from making good choices, that being healthy was an important marker of responsibility and morality, and that eating right was an especially important means of striving for health in both its biomedical and social aspects. As the discourse of alternative food promoted a normative experience of pleasure as essential to eating right, it recruited more of the individual into the overall duty to eat right. With this expansion, eating right was an increasingly salient social and moral duty that enlisted not only behaviors but the tastes, preferences, and subjectivity of the eater.

From Passive Victims to Active Consumers

As alternative food discourse redefined good food, it produced a new set of ideas about the good eater. In this context, being informed about nutrition and acting on that knowledge no longer amounted to the sum total of eating right. Instead, being a good eater entailed acting responsibly on knowledge about where food came from. It was about being a critical, active, responsible participant in the food system, rather than a passive consumer of industrial food. These dietary ideals reflected emerging notions of good citizenship. While domestic scientists intentionally promoted ideals that fit the demands of Progressive Era citizenship and wartime reformers explicitly linked eating right to good wartime citizenship, alternative food reformers advanced social ideals that were, perhaps more inadvertently, consistent with ideals of good citizenship shaped by the exigencies of neoliberalization. By 1980, the economic theory of neoliberalism, with its faith in free markets, property rights, and individual autonomy, had begun to reshape cultural notions of good citizenship. The good citizen was increasingly imagined as an autonomous, informed individual acting responsibly in his or her own self-interest, primarily through the market, as an educated consumer. Dovetailing with the new health consciousness, the ethos of neoliberalism shifted the burden of caring for the well-being of citizens from the state to the individual and recast health as a personal pursuit, responsibility, and duty.[36] As the burden of solving social problems and preserving the health of individuals shifted from the public to the private sector, alternative dietary ideals reinforced the increasingly important social values of personal responsibility and conscious consumption.

As alternative food reformers called for a new relationship with food, agriculture, and the food industry, they developed an image of an ideal eater who was active, informed, responsible, and both health- and pleasure-seeking. Unlike domestic scientists and World War II food reformers, who explicitly embraced emerging notions of good citizenship, alternative food reformers advocated a dietary ideal that was meant to be socially disruptive but subtly, and inadvertently, promoted some of the same values and characteristics that were part and parcel of neoliberal ideals of good citizenship. For example, books by Joan Gussow, the novelist Barbara Kingsolver, and Michael Pollan modeled and advocated informed, active involvement in food production as a social responsibility, moral duty, and a means of self-fulfillment. While their vision of good eating involved functioning as much as possible outside of the market, their message was easily interpreted as promoting the kind of educated, responsible consumption that was a hallmark of good neoliberal citizenship. In *This Organic Life* (2001), Gussow's memoir of her upstate New York garden and her year-round efforts to grow as much of her own food as possible, she described eating locally as "a morally responsible way to use the planet's resources." She explained that this kind of eating right was not about sacrificing pleasure, but about pursuing both responsibility and pleasure at the same time: "My peaches are among the many things that have convinced me that deliciousness is the best reason to eat food grown nearby and in season."[37] Barbara Kingsolver exemplified being an active, responsible good eater in *Animal, Vegetable, Miracle* (2007), her bestselling chronicle of a year in which she and her family strove to be independent of industrial agriculture, eating as locally as possible and growing much of their food themselves on a small farm in Appalachia. Like Gussow, Kingsolver celebrated the intertwined responsibility and pleasure of the enterprise, explaining, "Food is a rare moral arena in which the ethical choice is generally the one more likely to make you groan with pleasure."[38] Pollan also exemplified and advocated the active ideal, contrasting the deluded pleasures of the industrial meal to the authentic pleasures of the "hunted and gathered" one, in *Omnivore's Dilemma*. Pollan describes the meal he hunted, gathered, and grew himself as the "Perfect Meal" because "this labor- and thought-intensive dinner, enjoyed in the company of fellow foragers" gave him the chance to "eat in full consciousness of everything involved in feeding [him]self."[39] Each of these memoirs modeled and celebrated what it meant to be a good eater in the context of alternative food while subtly, and inadvertently, naturalizing what it meant to be a good citizen in the context of neoliberalization.

While Gussow, Kingsolver, and Pollan inspired readers with their adventures in informed, responsible, and pleasurable eating, Alice Waters set out to teach this version of eating right to children through the Edible Schoolyard, a gardening and cooking program at a public middle school in Berkeley. Waters was explicit that these lessons in eating right were meant to function as a pedagogy of good citizenship. The intent of the Edible Schoolyard, a model program that would eventually inspire many others like it, was to produce good eaters and good citizens by providing students with the interlinked experiences of knowledge, responsibility, and pleasure that were at the core of alternative food ideals. Waters's aim was to critique mainstream culture and provide an alternative through food, but the Edible Schoolyard was consistent with the political and social realities of neoliberalism in terms of both the social role it played and the qualities and characteristics it promoted as essential to good citizenship. The first phase of the process of neoliberalization, known as the roll-back phase, involved the dismantling of the welfare state.[40] The second phase, or the roll-out phase, was characterized by projects, like the Edible Schoolyard, that sought to address deficiencies in services, regulations, and social safety nets that were created by neoliberalization's rollbacks.[41] In their efforts to fill these gaps, advocates of such projects not infrequently reproduced neoliberal forms, practices, and subjects.[42] At the Edible Schoolyard, volunteers on the local level filled the gaps created by the rollbacks of neoliberalization and promoted social ideals that were consistent with the political-economic project of neoliberalism and the related demands of healthism.

The Edible Schoolyard project was launched in the mid-1990s and by the early twenty-first century had become both an icon of alternative food and a highly replicated model for similar projects across the nation (and beyond). Chez Panisse became a national sensation in the 1970s, and by the mid-1980s the restaurant was being hailed as "a revolution in American cooking."[43] But in the 1990s Waters's attention shifted to a different kind of revolution: the cascade of social change she believed could be touched off by changing people's eating habits. The Edible Schoolyard was reputed to have begun when Waters remarked on the deteriorating condition of the Martin Luther King Jr. Middle School in Berkeley in an interview and was shortly thereafter contacted by its principal. Influenced by her experience as a Montessori schoolteacher before opening Chez Panisse, Waters, like Ellen Richards, believed in the value of training the senses, muscles, and intellect of students through "practical life exercises."[44] Also inspired by the highly successful Garden Project at the San Francisco County Jail, in which inmates learned organic gardening, Waters began to imagine a similar social-reform project at the school, where 40 percent of students qualified for the federal free or reduced lunch program.[45]

As the vision for the garden was realized, beginning with the clearing of an abandoned asphalt lot adjacent to the school in December 1995, Waters formed the Chez Panisse Foundation to fund the project and others like it, and established a relationship with an ecologically oriented nonprofit, the Center for Ecoliteracy, which provided both additional funding and the intellectual basis for the curriculum.[46] Once the Edible Schoolyard was established, its influence spread through media exposure, an online presence, and advocacy that brought its principles to other schools and communities. An affiliate network launched in 2006 set out to prove that the program could succeed in a wide range of geographical and cultural environments. Described as the "backbone of our efforts" to "expand Alice Waters's vision for fostering hands-on learning, healthier food choices, and respect for one other, and the land," the program included an Edible Schoolyard at a New Orleans charter school, another at a charter school in Los Angeles, a project throughout the New York City public-school system, as well as programs in an upstate New York camp, a San Francisco boys and girls club, and a children's museum in Greensboro, North Carolina.[47] The Edible Schoolyard also provided resources for educators across the country interested in developing similar programs, including manuals, training workshops, and, starting in 2009, a summer academy.

Waters's interest in teaching the values and practices of alternative food to schoolchildren emerged directly from her conviction that teaching people to eat right could improve social life by cultivating good citizens. She believed that families were failing to provide the essential training for good citizenship offered by growing, preparing, and sharing food, and that the public schools had a critical role to play in rebuilding the social fabric by bringing those lessons back into the lives of children. Waters's convictions about the relationship between family mealtimes, social degradation, and the mandate of the public schools were strikingly similar to those espoused by Ellen Richards and other domestic scientists nearly a century earlier. Waters noted that "the family meal [had] undergone a steady devaluation" and argued that "public education must restore the daily ritual of the table in all of our children's lives."[48] In 1911, looking back on the social significance of the home-economics movement, Ellen Richards described the 1870s as a time when the "standard of the family table seemed to be deteriorating," and recalled that "careful observers of the social condition" saw more clearly than ever the "ethical value of the meeting place, around the common board, of young and old."[49]

For Waters, the table was such an important site for the training of good citizens that she called the family meal the "core curriculum of civilizing discourse" and described it as "a set of protocols that curb our natural savagery and our animal greed, and cultivate our capacity for sharing and thoughtfulness."[50] But work responsibilities, industrially produced alternatives to home-cooked meals, the distractions of media culture, and a frenetic pace of activity led many to eat alone or on the go instead of slowing down around a home-cooked meal with family and friends. Waters's concerns echoed those of Richards, who worried as early as 1895 that children were not learning to eat right at home: "The close parental watch which was formerly kept over children has weakened, and the child of today does pretty much as he pleases, even as to eating breakfast, taking lunches from home, or buying from the bakeshop."[51] Richards, who described home economics as "nothing less than an effort to save our social fabric from what seems inevitable disintegration," argued that public schools needed to step in to provide the third "R"—training for "right living."[52] One hundred years later Waters argued that teaching children good eating habits was even more important than the original "Rs." "We can do without reading and writing," she insisted, "but we certainly can't do without eating."[53]

At the Edible Schoolyard, lessons in the garden, kitchen, and classroom were designed to provide the interlinked experiences of knowledge, responsibility, and pleasure that would produce good citizens: people who took responsibility for their own health and the health of their communities, acted responsibly within the market as educated consumers, and made informed decisions in search of self-fulfillment. All students at the King School participated in classes in the garden, where they gained direct experience with where food came from, by weeding, turning compost, preparing beds, planting, and harvesting food for the kitchen (see figure 4.1). This knowledge was paired with pleasure, as students were given time for "foraging" in the garden and were encouraged to develop their senses by learning to enjoy fresh-picked strawberries, peas, and other garden produce. In the kitchen, students extended both their knowledge about where food came from and their pleasure in "good food" by learning to prepare the garden's harvest using their senses and a minimum of electric appliances. Lessons in the kitchen began with a presentation of the day's recipe, after which students prepared the recipes in small groups, tasting along the way. Once food was prepared, students were guided through a ritual of the table that was intended to socialize and civilize (see figure 4.2). They set tables with cloths, plates, silverware, and fresh flowers, and sat

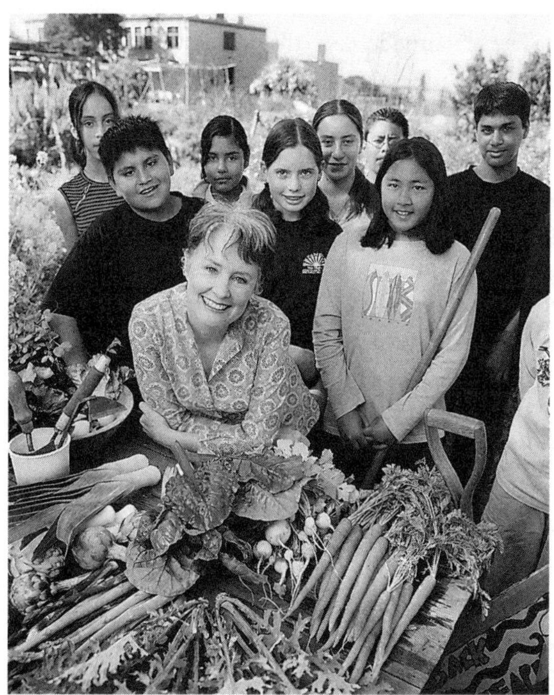

FIGURE 4.1 • Alice Waters with students and produce at the Edible Schoolyard. Photo courtesy of the Edible Schoolyard Project.

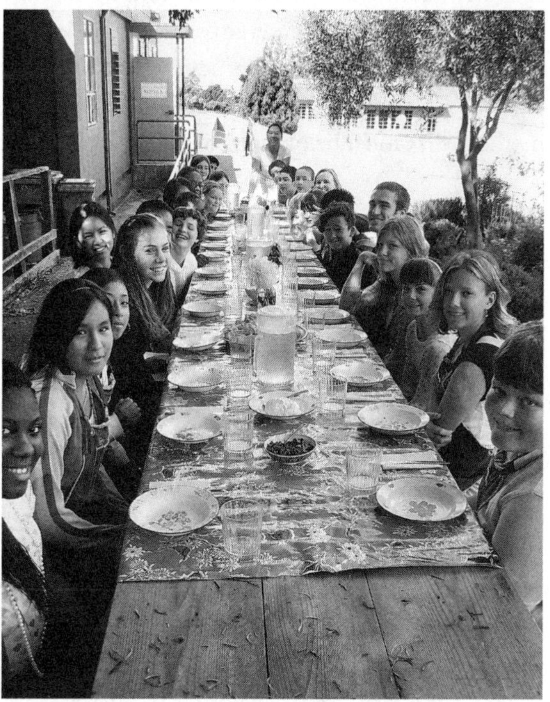

FIGURE 4.2 • Mealtime at the Edible Schoolyard as a civilizing, socializing ritual. Photo courtesy of the Edible Schoolyard Project.

down to eat and talk. The staff made sure that mealtime conversation fulfilled its social purpose by creating "Question Cards" to stimulate meaningful conversation.[54]

Despite Waters's avowedly anticonsumerist stance, the aims of the Edible Schoolyard reinforced the neoliberal notion that good citizenship was practiced through responsible consumption. Training ethical citizens was approached as a matter of teaching students to find sensual pleasures in beautiful foods and embrace a moral obligation to support sustainable agriculture and the well-being of the planet by consuming responsibly. As Waters explained to President Clinton in the early years of the Edible Schoolyard, she believed that similar programs should be in every school in order to demonstrate "to a new generation of citizens how our decisions about food affect the survival of us all, and how eating can become a consuming habit that can give us pleasure every day of our lives," while also creating "a binding sense of social responsibility."[55] Lessons in both the garden and the kitchen cultivated skills related to consumer choice, while the overarching message of the Edible Schoolyard explicitly conflated those skills with good citizenship.[56] As Julie Guthman and Patricia Allen argue, this conflation is a "key neoliberal conceit" that works against the social change many activists would like to see emerge by absolving "people of the need to do anything else beyond selecting products for purchase" and reinforcing "the idea that social change is simply a matter of individual will rather than something that must be organized and struggled over in collectivities."[57]

The lessons of the Edible Schoolyard also reflected the exponential expansion in the obligation of personal responsibility as a core component of good citizenship that occurred within the context of neoliberalization. By the end of the twentieth century, the sense of the scale and scope of environmental and health risks had become far greater than ever before, and individuals were increasingly expected to mitigate those risks by making healthy and responsible choices.[58] In comparison to the domestic-science view of dietary choices as impacting municipalities, for example, in the early twenty-first century dietary reformers preached that eating habits had an impact far beyond the immediate environment in which they took place. Threats to individuals and communities were now broadened to the planet and the species, and also well into the future. For students of the Edible Schoolyard, and the good eaters of the alternative food movement more generally, eating right meant taking personal responsibility for threats to an "environment" that was conceived with essentially no constraints of time (into the perpetual future) or of space (the planet and beyond). This meant that the discourse of alternative food expanded the purview of dietary reform in not one but two ways: it extended the meaning of eating right deeper into the self by harnessing rather than repressing pleasure, while it also expanded the spatial and temporal sphere of the social responsibility and moral duty of eating right into, essentially, infinity.

The Healthy Middle Class and the Cheap, Fast Other

The alternative food discourse of dietary reform increased the moral freight of eating right by advocating ethical rather than quantitative norms, emphasizing personal responsibility for societal well-being, and expanding the realm of responsibility infinitely. It also produced a moralized class hierarchy that, because of this increased moral freight, was especially significant. Domestic scientists established eating right as an important pursuit for members of the middle class wishing to identify themselves as race saviors rather than race destroyers and as a way by which members of the "thinking classes" could distinguish themselves from those in the laboring class, who seemed to lack the intelligence and will to eat what was good for them rather than what they liked. Wartime reformers presented a less divided portrait of American society, but nonetheless reconfirmed existing ideas about health as the purview of the middle class by claiming that the diets of defense workers and their families presented a particularly grave threat to the war effort and were especially difficult to improve because of worker "indifference" to nutrition. Dietary thinking in the late twentieth century built on the established relationship between the middle class, health, and dietary health. But dietary talk may have had a greater impact on the construction of class at this time than at any other point in the history of modern dietary reform because health practices had become more significant to identity and subjectivity, eating habits were considered more central to health, and individuals bore such an extensive burden of responsibility for not only their own health but also the health of the social order, the environment, the planet, and the future.

Beginning in the 1970s, economic and cultural shifts caused a fragmenting of the middle class that brought into being an upper middle class distinguished in part by its interest in health, fitness, and food. Crawford explains that health reemerged as a major preoccupation for the American middle class in the late 1970s. An increasing sense of health risks alongside growing concerns about the social and economic viability of the middle class led many to new health and fitness regimes. Incomes were falling, the cost of maintaining a middle-class lifestyle was rising, workplace competition was heating up, and, for many, fitness regimes provided a way to practice and perform qualities of self that might help to protect and preserve status.[59] But it was primarily among the upper strata of the fragmenting middle class that health became a major preoccupation in the late twentieth century. The economic stresses of the 1970s precipitated a polarization in wealth between lower and upper levels of the middle class, as manufacturing jobs disappeared or were replaced with lower-paying service jobs. The blue-collar middle class began losing ground around 1977–78, but as Belasco notes, in the mid-1970s market research—which often served "as an early warning system for emerging tendencies"—had begun to detect a separation of the middle class into two groups: "upscale/'healthy'" and "downscale/'regular.'" As Belasco explains, marketers found that more educated, affluent members of the middle class were more likely to be interested in RDAs, more likely to read food labels, and more concerned about additives in their food. Wealthier households, one study found, "were most likely to buy foods 'highly correlated with nutritional concern.'"[60] The findings remained consistent through the 1980s, with the less affluent deemed "less careful" about how they ate compared to "the upper 40 percent," who were considered "health conscious." As Belasco points out, the "national obsession" with dietary health widely reported in the media throughout the 1980s was taking place primarily among this "upper 40 percent."[61] And it was these health-conscious and food-focused Americans of the upper middle class who, from the mid-1990s onward, visited Chez Panisse and bought Alice Waters's cookbooks, supported the Edible Schoolyard and started programs like it in their own schools, read Michael Pollan and Barbara Kingsolver, and avidly pursued eating right in its new ecological-ethical iteration.

The alternative food ethos of dietary health reinforced the distinction between the "upper 40 percent" and the "less careful" other by insisting that essential for a "good diet" were two ingredients likely to be more available to the more affluent strata of the middle class: time and money. A fundamental argument of the alternative food movement was that eating right meant refusing the cheap conveniences of mass-produced foods and spending more money on ingredients and more time preparing and enjoying them. Pollan, for example, argued that unreasonable expectations for cheap food were created by an unhealthy, unsustainable food system and that Americans could and should pay more—in both time and money—for food. He pointed out that Americans spent a smaller percentage of their income on food than people in any other industrialized society and argued that most could afford to spend more on food: "Maybe 25 percent of the people in this country can't move toward a diet that's more local and organic. . . . The other people are making a judgment about priorities."[62] Pointing to the amount of time and money Americans found to spend on the Internet in the last decade, he reasoned that for most people paying more for food was "less a matter of ability than priority."[63] Furthermore, he conjectured, it might be a good idea for people to spend more and eat less; spending more on smaller quantities of higher-quality food could bring down obesity rates and reign in the health-care costs that soared—not coincidently—as food spending declined.[64]

Waters also frequently argued that eating right was a matter of making the choice to spend more time and money on food. She said that Americans spent a "pitifully small fraction of their income on food" and could double what they currently spent "and still have plenty left over."[65] She urged people to spend more for organics, noting that there were hidden costs in cheap food that were paid for in farm subsidies, Middle Eastern oil, depleted soil, and health consequences.[66] Eating right also meant carefully choosing, preparing, serving, and savoring food, rather than simply fueling up on food prepared by strangers. We should all know, Waters reminded, "anything worth doing takes time."[67] She argued that it was a mistake to think that "no fuss, no mess, and no preparation time are good things." Trying to save time by not cooking or shopping, she explained, we miss out on one of the "few worthwhile pleasures in life—not in getting away from work but in doing good work that means something."[68]

Advocating a way of eating that was out of reach for so many Americans invited frequent charges of elitism against Waters, Pollan, and the movement in general. Critics argued that the ideals of the alternative food movement were unrealistic, inequitable, and therefore an ineffective response to the problems in the American food system they attempted to solve. They said that the vision was patently elitist, accessible only to the wealthy despite the reformers' insistence that it should be otherwise.[69] Critics pointed to the irony of the hungry and homeless who panhandled outside of Chez Panisse, the insensitivity of arguing that people should be willing to pay more for food, and the "stigma of elitism" that the movement accrued when it failed to acknowledge that most people cannot afford to eat fresh, local food.[70]

As frequent targets of the elitism critique, Waters and Pollan both insisted that ultimately their work was about making eating right more accessible. In a *60 Minutes* profile of Waters, Lesley Stahl gave Waters a chance to respond to the charge that "Alice Waters is self-righteous and elitist." Waters said, "I feel that good food should be a right and not a privilege and it needs to be without pesticides and herbicides. And everybody deserves this food. And that's not elitist."[71] But in the end the interview only led to more charges of elitism.[72] Later in the segment, as she made the rounds at a farmers market with Waters, Stahl noticed grapes selling for $4 a pound and brought up the common complaint about how expensive organic food is. Waters responded with a comment that perfectly exhibited the insensitivity toward the real constraints that many people face, with its subtle classism and racism, that enflamed her critics: "We make decisions everyday about what we're going to eat," she said. "And some people want to buy Nike shoes—two pairs—and other people want to eat Bronx grapes, and nourish themselves. I pay a little extra, but this is what I want to do."[73] Pollan's reaction to charges of elitism revolved around the argument that eating well was elitist only because of misguided government policies that made it so. In a 2006 *New York Times* blog post he explained, "Our tax dollars are the reason that the cheapest calories in the market are the least healthy ones," and he argued for farm policies that would "right this imbalance" so that eating well would no longer be "elitist."[74] Pollan also explained that the movement was indeed started by elites who had the time and resources to put toward it, just like many U.S. social movements (abolition, suffrage, etc.) and that "to damn a political and social movement because the people who started it are well-to-do seems to me not all that damning. If the food movement is still dominated by the elite in 20 years, I think that will be damning."[75]

Both the charges of elitism levied against the alternative food movement and these defenses against them focused on problems of accessibility and equitability. But the exclusivity of these ideals was significant and problematic not only because a good diet was not available to the poor but also because of the historical interplay between eating habits, subjectivity, and status. The ideals of alternative food, like those of other modern dietary movements, contributed to the construction and naturalization of class and established, in effect, a hierarchy of morality and responsibility that legitimized the status of the healthy (upper) middle class, once again, in contrast to the "unhealthy other." Crawford argues that from the 1970s onward in the context of "rapidly expanding mandates for healthy behavior" and increasing focus on prevention, the health / illness distinction came to connote, ever more so, the distinction between the deserving and the defective. This dynamic increased the healthy person's investment in maintaining the distinction between themselves and those perceived as "unhealthy," leading to "a social distancing from the 'unhealthy,' a further stereotyping of already stigmatized groups who then, because of their 'irresponsible' habits, are confirmed in their otherness."[76]

Whether or not people could assume the practices of eating right as defined by alternative food reformers mattered in terms of class because of the historical relationship between dietary ideals and social ideals that this book has traced so far, and particularly so because the social stakes related to health practices in general were so high at the turn of the millennium. But whether or not people could assume the practices of eating right may have mattered even more so because of the explicit argument that alternative food reformers made about eating habits as an expression of values and ethics. Because this dietary reform movement focused on transmitting ethics rather than quantitative norms of a good diet, it produced a much more explicit set of ideas about the meaning of eating right in relation to individual morality. The ethical and moral dimensions of eating habits were overtly central to the philosophy. A moral hierarchy of good and bad eaters was constructed and affirmed every time a well-meaning reformer described the contrast between the responsible, moral pleasure of eating right and the delusional, destructive, habits of industrial eaters. If the good eater was motivated by knowledge about the origins of food to make careful choices about what to eat that would benefit society and the environment, the bad eater passively and ignorantly indulged in destructive cheap conveniences.

For many alternative food reformers, fast food was the pinnacle, or nadir, of thoughtless industrial eating. The critique of fast food and fast-food eaters was particularly striking in its class implications because of the accessibility and appeal of fast food for people facing scarcities of time, wealth, and access to fresh produce. For example, in a 1990 essay Frances Moore Lappé, a major figure in both the countercuisine and alternative food, lamented the cheap pleasures of fast food: "Since human beings are adaptable creatures, we become convinced that . . . heating processed food in a microwave oven is cooking, and that fast-food and chain restaurants are an adequate substitute for the pleasure, community, and solace that traditional restaurant and family meals once gave us."[77] In a similar vein, Kingsolver bemoaned the immediate appeal of fast food: "Eating preprocessed or fast food can look like salvation in the short run, until we start losing what real mealtimes give to a family: civility, economy and health."[78] And she made clear that cooking, in contrast, was a more moral, responsible choice: "Cooking is good citizenship. It's the only way to get serious about putting locally raised foods into your diet, which keeps farmland healthy and grocery money in the neighborhood."[79]

Waters frequently used "fast food" to stand in for bad food and described an entire set of (bad) values associated with and fostered by eating cheap, fast food. "When you buy fast food," she claimed, "you get fast food values."[80] According to Waters, she came up with the idea of "fast food values" after reading Schlosser's *Fast Food Nation*. The book caused her to consider what happened to the moral fiber of American children when they were exposed to fast food. "What lessons," she asked, "do they absorb by osmosis when they eat a happy meal? What are the values that fast food inculcates in them?"[81] Waters identified a set of values that she believed were promoted by the consumption of fast food and had come to permeate American culture: food is "cheap and abundant" and "abundance is permanent"; "resources are infinite so it's perfectly okay to waste"; eating is about "fueling up" quickly; "it doesn't matter where the food actually comes from"; "work is to be avoided at all costs."[82] Eating fast food was not just bad for individual health, but bad for communities, bad for the earth, immoral.

Waters presented the choice between fast food and its alternative, slow food, as a profoundly moral one with real consequences in terms of either improving or degrading the world. She explained in a 2002 interview that we all have to eat to live and that "we can do that in a very destructive way, destroying not only ourselves but the land around us, or we can do it in a very conscious, pleasurable way."[83] When people buy fast food, she explained, they may think that they are getting off with only a "halfway-toxic hamburger, but it's a whole lot more than that."[84] She argued that choosing to eat mass-produced fast food supported "a network of supply and demand that is destroying local communities and traditional ways of life all over the world."[85] In contrast, Waters described eating fresh food that was locally grown by farmers who took care of the earth as contributing "to the health and stability of local agriculture and local communities."[86] While fast food inculcated a set of values that "[flew] in the face of thousands of years of human experience," Waters argued that slow food could teach people "all the things that really matter—care, beauty, concentration, discernment, sensuality—all the best that humans are capable of."[87] Slow-food eaters were characterized as connecting with a noble past and making thoughtful, conscious choices that enhanced both personal fulfillment and social well-being. Fast-food eaters were portrayed as just the opposite: unthinking dupes, whose lack of "consciousness" kept them trapped in irresponsible habits and drawn to immoral pleasures.

The opposition between fast and slow food, good and bad eaters, was a way for individuals to identify themselves and assess others. For many people who could afford to spend more time and money to eat right, doing so became a way of expressing their values, ethics, and morality in contrast to those who were both bad eaters and bad subjects. Deborah Lupton documented a similar situation in Australia, where she conducted interviews with people about their food preference. She found that for many people eating was "a secular means of attributing meaning and value to everyday practices." Eating right—eating slow, natural, authentic, fresh, local food—provided a means by which to both express and assess morality as, in part, a function of conscious, thoughtful, reflexive consumption. Every mouthful of food, she found, served as a "politico-moral statement."[88] Fast food and slow food became not only material, but also moral, opposites.[89]

Working through the fast-slow opposition, the discourse of alternative food naturalized a distinctly moralized hierarchy of class. The binary was meaningful in part because fast-food eating was more prevalent among those in the lower classes due to the affordable calories and convenience it offered, often in neighborhoods with few alternatives, and also because it was more symbolically associated with people of color and the poor, even though fast food was eaten by Americans across the social and economic spectrum. In one speech, Waters herself pointed out that fast-food eating was "pervasive (especially in poor communities)."[90] But because the social construction of class was obscured, bad eating habits seemed more like evidence of character weakness that justified lower-class status, rather than the result of the combination of factors—including occupation, income, and neighborhood—that constituted class.

This naturalization of class was reinforced by reformers ignoring constraints on consumption choices that were imposed neither by a lack of knowledge nor by a failure of reflexive subjectivity, but rather by the complex of factors that also constitute class. Pollan reasoned that choosing bad food was more often than not simply a matter of having the wrong priorities—spending money on broadband and television instead of on grass-fed beef, pastured eggs, and unprocessed foods that are ideally both local and organic.[91] Waters explicitly described eating right as a choice that people were free to make, "without anyone's permission and without anyone's help."[92] In a 2001 interview she was asked to comment on the irony of homeless and hungry people panhandling outside of Chez Panisse. Her response showed the extent of her conviction that eating right was simply a matter of having the right kind of knowledge, as well as her tendency to ignore financial realities and other constraints (such as lacking a home in which to bathe or cook) that might influence eating habits. To her, the presence of panhandlers outside of Chez Panisse underscored the urgency of helping people "to understand the relationship of food to their lives. To understand, very early, how to take care of themselves." A person educated to understand the real social and ethical value of slow food, Waters assumed, would make the kind of choices that she herself made, and she, for one, "would rather split a calzone and a large green salad and have a glass of wine for $10 a person in the lower-priced Café Panisse [above Chez Panisse] than fill [her] face for $7.50 at some cheap joint."[93]

This moralized class hierarchy was also naturalized by the rhetoric that alternative dietary reformers used to legitimize their dietary ideals. For other modern dietary reformers, legitimacy came from the authority of science, the seeming objectivity of which made their ideals of a good diet seem natural, even inevitable, in spite of the fact that they reflected middle-class preferences and served middle-class interests. Alternative dietary ideals, based on a refusal of scientific rationality, were instead made to seem irrefutably true through the language of universality, history, and tradition. Reformers assumed, for example, a certain universality of taste, as if a preference for "good food" were somehow inherent. Waters, in particular, believed that the senses were a universal guide that, if given the chance, would lead everyone to follow the norms she advocated.[94] In a 2003 speech, for example, she described the senses as "the great equalizer" and celebrated the beauty of a sensory education that leaves you "defenseless against your better nature."[95] Pollan also frequently reinforced the perception that the senses were a universal guide that, if not intercepted by the Nutritional Industrial Complex, would lead everyone to delight in good food. Also evoking other apparently indisputable grounds, he explained, "Most of what we need to know about how to eat we already know, or once did, until we allowed the nutrition experts and the advertisers to shape our confidence in common sense, tradition, the testimony of our senses, and the wisdom of our mothers and grandmothers."[96] Proponents frequently claimed authority through a connection to history and tradition, asserting that there was nothing new about their ideas and suggesting that they simply represented a return to a better past. Waters portrayed bad eating habits ("fast food and its attendant values") as an affront to history and tradition, and described her work as nothing more than being "true to a philosophy of food that has been part of the fabric of life since the beginning of time."[97] Eating seasonally, locally, and organically, she explained, was "a return to traditional values of the most fundamental kind."[98] Together, these strategies, whether intentionally or unintentionally, presented alternative thinking about food and the moralized class hierarchy it instantiated as perfectly natural.

ALTERNATIVE FOOD was in some senses a liberating reappraisal of convention, offering people a whole new way of thinking about what made food "good" that encouraged critical distance from nutrition and rejection of the industrial food system and all it stood for. It promoted a sense of connection that people clearly craved and a relationship with "nature" that brought meaning and solace to lives that were often experienced as too hectic, too urban, and too technological. This was a dietary ideal that celebrated sensuality, intuition, and tradition, ways of relating to food that had no place in the calculations of nutrition. And it not only endorsed, but also promoted pleasure. Pleasure in cooking, eating, and sharing food were now part of the "prescription" for eating right.

Despite all of this, alternative food does not read as a radical departure within the history of dietary reform. It foregrounded the ethics of eating right, celebrating the ways in which choosing good food was a moral act, but alternative food provided rules about what to eat that were no less normalizing than those prescribed by nutrition and maybe even more so. The celebration of pleasure may have made eating right more fun, but it meant that compliance required not only doing but also feeling certain things: eating right now mandated the enjoyment of eating right. Against the backdrop of social changes that made health and diet more significant than ever before, the focus on ethics actually heightened the moral valence of eating right within alternative food, creating higher stakes for good and bad eating than in previous eras. Alternative food produced trenchant critiques of the dietary status quo and much-needed public dialogue about the ethics of the industrial system of food production, but it wielded its own moral force with little self-awareness or critique.

All of this took place alongside the emergence of obesity as a health problem, national crisis, and target for reform. Distinctly biomedical in its orientation, the antiobesity movement emphasized the empirical aspects of nutrition, but capitalized on and enhanced its moral and social valence. These two simultaneous reform movements were both contradictory and complementary. In some sense they pulled in opposite directions, but their similarities and convergences were striking. They occasionally overlapped in concern, strategy, and focus. Perhaps more important, they worked together to establish a new common sense around eating right as a morally loaded, socially significant factor in modern American life.

FIVE

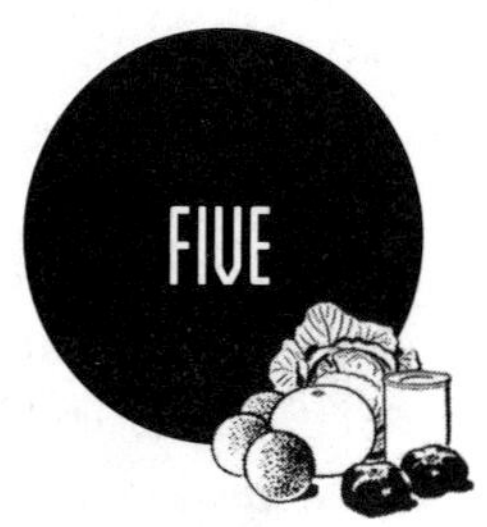

THINNESS AS HEALTH, SELF-CONTROL, AND CITIZENSHIP

In April 2009 a group of fifth-grade students from a nearby public school spent an afternoon at the White House planting vegetable seeds on the South Lawn. First Lady Michelle Obama proudly welcomed them to what she called the White House Kitchen Garden, which by harvest time would be renamed the First Lady's Garden at the White House. Naming aside, the mission of the garden was clear: to educate students, their families, and the public about eating right. The last time food had been grown on the White House Lawn was in a victory garden installed by Eleanor Roosevelt in 1943 to inspire the nation at war. News coverage of the Obama garden periodically noted that it was making a similar political point, sending a message about the social importance of growing and eating good food.[1] The twenty-five varieties of fruits, vegetables, and herbs planted from heirloom seeds in the Obama's 1,100-square-foot garden represented a major transformation in the cultural politics of dietary health since the end of the Great War and was celebrated as a major victory for the alternative food movement. Though many in the blogosphere disagreed, the mass media credited Alice Waters, with ABC News noting, "Alice Waters, the nation's leading advocate for sustainable agriculture, has been pushing the Obamas to take the lead on food policy and plant a garden," and the Associated Press calling the White House Garden "a dream of noted California chef Alice Waters, considered a leader in the movement to encourage consumption of locally grown, organic food."[2] But while the garden championed an ecological understanding of good food, it also reified a biomedical view of health and a nutritional concept of eating right. It represented a convergence of alternative food with another major dietary reform movement: the war against obesity.

A few months after the garden was planted, Michelle Obama addressed a crowd of middle-school children (and the press) at a harvest party. She congratulated the children for picking lettuce, shelling peas, cooking chicken and brown rice, and preparing a delicious dressing for the salad. But before the children got to sit down to enjoy their meal, she explained, she wanted to make sure that everyone understood why they were there. Why did the garden matter to the First Lady? What was it supposed to mean to the American people? According to Obama, the garden was a fun way for the students to learn to try different things, and to experience the pleasures of produce that tasted better because it was fresh and locally grown. Her reason for engaging students in the pleasures of good food, however, was not simply to cultivate ethical eaters, but also to help combat the infamous obesity epidemic. According to Obama, the First Lady's Garden was a "fun and interesting way to talk to kids about health and nutrition" at a time when "nearly a third of the children in this country [were] either overweight or obese": "Too many kids," she stated, "are consuming high-calorie foods with low nutritional value, and they are not getting enough exercise."[3] She explained that the idea for the garden came from her own experience feeding her daughters and, as a working mother, having to rely on eating out or ordering pizza a few times a week. After the girls' pediatrician "raised a red flag" because they were gaining weight, Obama said she started thinking more about nutrition and wanted to bring what she had learned to "a broader base of people" by planting a vegetable garden on the South Lawn of the White House.[4] At the harvest party, she said her goal was to encourage kids to eat better and to educate their families "about how to eat in a healthier way."[5]

The First Lady's Garden drew on two distinct meanings of dietary health and two very different dietary-reform movements that by the early years of the twenty-first century had become increasingly interrelated. On the one hand, the garden evoked the ethos of alternative food, establishing a model for good-food citizenship that entailed using the senses to reconnect with food, knowing where food came from, and taking pleasure in fresh, local, sustainably produced fruits and vegetables. On the other hand, it exemplified the logic of the campaign against obesity, which conceived of dietary health in a very different way. The garden represented a convergence of these two modes of thinking about eating right that was already evident in various alternative food undertakings that invoked obesity as proof that the industrial food system was bad for people and a primary reason that alternatives, such as farm-to-school programs, were desperately needed.[6] Articulating this juncture, Waters described the obesity epidemic as "a symptom of a deeper issue: how fast food and industrial agriculture are destroying the environment and our culture."[7] Pollan made these links famous in his *New York Times Magazine* article "The (Agri)Cultural Contradictions of Obesity" and in his best-selling book *In Defense of Food*, in which he blamed obesity on agricultural policies that promoted overproduction and, therefore, overconsumption.[8] Yet the campaign against obesity emphasized the biomedical and empirical aspects of nutrition that alternative food frequently defined itself against and obscured the moral dimensions of dietary health that alternative food championed.

Building on the argument that dietary advice is always both empirical and ethical, I explore those moral dimensions, arguing that like other dietary-reform movements, the campaign against obesity expressed social ideals related to notions of good citizenship and established a moralized dietary hierarchy that served to delineate unstable social boundaries. I examine the reorientation of the discourse of dietary health around body size and the persistent equivalence between thinness and self-control within the discourse of obesity, suggesting that both contributed to the major expansion in the scope and social significance of dietary reform that we have already seen. In so doing I explain why, in the context of obesity, the consequences of being a "bad eater" were more serious than ever before.

Unlike other dietary-reform movements I have examined, the campaign against obesity generated stigma that severely compromised the life chances of those it purported to help. Because of this it has also generated a far more robust countermovement than the other movements I have discussed. Among fat-acceptance activists and fat-studies scholars who challenge the factual premise of the so-called obesity epidemic and rigorously critique the negative social effects of antiobesity discourse, *obesity* is a contested term. It is understood to medicalize a form of human diversity and do violence to fat people, and it is therefore usually avoided or placed in scare quotes.[9] Though I consider this book, and especially this chapter, to be fat-studies scholarship, I use the terms *obesity* and *overweight* without scare quotes throughout. I trust the reader to understand by this point that I consider all forms of dietary discourse social constructions that have the potential to do violence to "bad eaters." I treat the term *obesity* no differently than I treat the term *hidden hunger*, for example. Antiobesity discourse is far more virulent in its social effects than are other dietary-reform movements, and *obesity* is therefore a far more potent term than are others used to describe dietary dangers, but the larger point of this book is to help make sense of how this came to be by showing that antiobesity discourse shares a common history with other modern dietary-reform movements that have capitalized on the empirical and ethical aspects of nutrition.

Alarming Expansions: Body Size and the Purview of Dietary Health

From a certain perspective, the campaign against obesity was unrecognizable as a dietary-reform campaign. Its reform message was diffuse in two key senses: it emanated from locations beyond nutrition and public health, and it focused broadly on a range of behaviors that transcended eating habits. Though clearly inseparable from concerns about the relationship between diet and health, its core message—that people needed to either attain or maintain a "healthy weight"—was not exactly dietary advice. Despite these qualities—or, more accurately, because of them—the antiobesity campaign was in fact a manifestation of modern dietary reform that took its logic to the extreme. In the context of postwar changes in the culture of health, the amount and kind of cultural work that dietary-reform movements could do intensified significantly. The diffuse and complex nature of the antiobesity campaign capitalized on the new significance of dietary health, extending the cultural reach and social impact of dietary discourse as each of the movements examined here has done. Its focus on body ideals transferred the cultural politics of eating right to the visible language of the body and to a wider range of behaviors than ever before, thus intensifying the stigma for "bad eaters" and bringing more aspects of daily life under the influence of "dietary" reform efforts. The fact that obesity was ultimately declared an "epidemic" and sometimes even referred to as a "global pandemic" attests to the way in which this dietary crisis exceeded the definitional and spatial boundaries of dietary reform that were established at the beginning of the twentieth century.

By the time a national epidemic of obesity was officially declared by the U.S. government, in 2001, the discourse of obesity as a social and dietary crisis was nearly half a century old, and extremely complex. Efforts to combat obesity were not centrally organized by the federal government as the National Nutrition Program had been, though the federal government did take part in and sometimes instigate antiobesity reform efforts. Neither was the antiobesity reform effort a grassroots movement championed by charismatic leaders, as was the alternative food movement. Instead, the antiobesity campaign comprised a vast and ever-growing array of programs and perspectives initiated and advanced by industry, academics, medical and public-health practitioners, the press, and the government. As I define the antiobesity-reform movement, it encompassed all manner of efforts to persuade, instruct, alarm, and assist Americans with the goal of reducing the incidence of overweight and obesity across the population; among these efforts were films and television shows, diet books, research studies, newspaper and magazine articles, nutrition and fitness campaigns, and federal initiatives. Unlike in the other movements I have examined, many of the players in this campaign stood to profit from defining obesity as health crisis. Weight-loss companies (e.g., Weight Watchers, Jenny Craig, Slim-Fast), authors and publishers of diet books, weight-loss doctors and surgeons, government health agencies, and even academic researchers and scientists all benefited from defining obesity as a disease that required treatment and reform.[10] By 2011 a sixty-billion-dollar-a-year industry thrived on the problem that obesity posed for Americans.[11] Although diet and weight-loss industries were remarkably ineffective (the failure rate for sustained weight loss was reported to be about 90–95 percent), they remained incredibly profitable. During the last fifty years, and particularly since the mid-1990s, diet and weight-loss industries also dramatically increased their influence over the federal government's public-health-related decision-making and played a hand in intensifying concerns about obesity from which they also profited.[12]

Abigail Saguy and Kevin Riley identify four sets of claimants "engaged in framing contests over the nature and consequences of excess body weight."[13] Two of these groups—antiobesity researchers and antiobesity activists—drove the language and logic of the reform movement I identify and analyze here. Antiobesity researchers studied obesity and argued that was an urgent health crisis. They were scientists from a variety of backgrounds, including but not limited to nutrition, and their work informed most media reporting on obesity. Saguy and Riley define antiobesity activists as "people committed to the antiobesity movement who do not do primary research, but who are involved in fighting obesity in other ways"; they were individuals who publicly argued that obesity deserved public intervention, research funding, and private action in any number of ways, including writing books, making films, and local advocacy.[14] On the other hand, "fat acceptance" activists and researchers rejected the very premise of the antiobesity campaign. They argued that fatness was a form of body diversity that should be respected, not changed, and insisted that focusing on obesity distracted attention from more important health problems while subjecting the targets of reform to prejudice and oppression.[15] From their perspective, the antiobesity campaign, predicated on the fallacious construction of obesity as a health problem, posed a far greater problem than did obesity itself.

The crisis of the late twentieth century and early twenty-first known as the "obesity epidemic" is widely believed to have begun in the mid-1990s with two reports that enflamed existing concerns about the rate at which population weights were increasing. But the conceptual link between weight and mortality that fueled and justified those concerns had been established in the immediate postwar period. The notion of obesity as an aesthetic, moral, and medical problem had existed since the early twentieth century, but the postwar period saw a major intensification of concern among the public, the press, and medical professionals.[16] It was during the years after World War II that the nutrition and public-health community reoriented itself around weight as a primary concern, that a consensus began to form around obesity as a medical problem, and that the notion that obesity posed a major threat to the well-being of individuals and the nation itself surfaced. Like the other dietary crises studied here, obesity was produced as a problem at the intersection of science and culture.

Efforts in the insurance industry to identify factors that correlated to early death, and therefore increased costs for the industry, motivated much of the research on obesity during the postwar period (and prior to it), but widespread public alarm about weight was inseparable from cultural concerns about the postwar lifestyle. The idea of obesity as a major national health crisis crystallized in the early 1950s in part due to a 1951 a

MetLife study that confirmed a significant relationship between weight and mortality, and validated the notion that there existed an ideal weight for being healthy.[17] There were serious flaws in the methods used to conduct these studies, but the results soon "came to be regarded as gospel," and medical professionals declared obesity America's leading health problem.[18] By 1950, obesity had already been called the "greatest single hazard to human life in the nation today" in the pages of the *New York Times*.[19] In 1952 excess body fat was referred to as a "devastating nutritional disorder" and declared the nation's "primary public health problem."[20]

These concerns about dietary health were fundamentally inseparable from larger cultural concerns about the impact of postwar affluence and leisure on the American character. An article published in the *New York Times* in 1950 explained that obesity was becoming a national problem in large part because of "mechanical improvements" and declared that "Americans [were] getting fat on too much food and too little work."[21] Another article complained that too many families were taking pride in overeating because it proved that they had "the affluence to be overfed."[22] The idea of obesity as a threat to the health and character of Americans intensified as MetLife reduced the weight range considered healthy throughout the postwar years. In 1942 the MetLife height-weight table determined that a man of average build should weigh between 145 and 156 pounds, but by 1959 he was expected to weigh between 138 and 152.[23] This lowered the "healthy weight" to about 10–15 percent below the national average, increasing overnight the number of people deemed unhealthy in America and laying the foundation for a surge in concern about obesity as the public-health community turned its attention to chronic diseases in the 1960s and 1970s.[24]

Concern about the relationship between diet, chronic disease, and obesity converged in the late 1960s to produce a new nutritional paradigm and a new sense of what it meant to eat right. A prominent nutritionist later recalled that after the war, the nutrition community recognized that the major vitamin-deficiency diseases had for the most part been vanquished. He and his colleagues worried briefly about the relevance of their field before it was "rescued by obesity" and the beginning of the "chronic disease era."[25] Ironically, national concern about obesity as a health problem escalated as a result of an effort to wage a "war against hunger." A series of hearings on poverty and malnutrition revealed that research into vitamins had been exhausted and that chronic diseases offered a new area of possibility for nutritional improvements.[26] The 1969 White House Conference on Food, Nutrition and Health was a turning point. The conference opened with a reconfirmation of the MetLife position that obesity was a real health problem clearly related to mortality.[27] Experts discussed both deficiency diseases and "the health problems of adults in affluent society—the degenerative diseases of middle age," which they determined were caused largely by "unwise" food choices.[28] Finally, the conference produced the first significantly revised dietary recommendations since the first RDAs were launched, on the eve of World War II. Among them were the suggestions to eat less of those foods containing too many calories and too much fat, cholesterol, salt, sugar, and alcohol.[29]

This new set of guidelines signaled a major change from earlier dietary advice, which focused on getting Americans to eat more health-promoting foods such as the vitamin-rich "protective foods" touted by war-era reformers. At the heart of the new nutritional paradigm, named "negative nutrition" by Belasco, was the idea that some foods could contribute to or cause chronic diseases, especially if consumed in large quantities, and should be avoided or eaten sparingly.[30] Though obesity was not a disease in the usual sense of the term, as the nutrition paradigm shifted toward negative nutrition, obesity was increasingly included among the chronic diseases that were considered linked to diet. In the early 1970s a series of hearings staged by the Select Committee on Nutrition and Human Needs focused national attention on the emerging paradigm of negative nutrition by highlighting the perils of overconsumption and the link between diet and obesity, diabetes, and heart disease.[31]

While there was a history of dieting and aesthetic preferences for slimness in America dating back to about the turn of the century, from the 1950s onward an increasing number of Americans began to worry about their weight. The growing focus of the medical community on obesity as a health problem was due in part to patients' ongoing requests for weight-loss advice. A conflation of science with cultural norms, a convergence of discovery and belief, caused doctors to focus on weight as an issue and endorse ever-decreasing recommended weights.[32] Polls show that concern about the problem of weight increased rapidly between the 1950s and the early 1970s, with the percentages of people who considered themselves overweight and of those dieting to lose weight soaring. The biggest changes were seen among women. In 1959, 21 percent of women judged themselves overweight and 14 percent were dieting; by 1973, 55 percent judged themselves overweight and 49 percent were trying to lose weight.[33] But from the perspective of the mid-1990s, when concern about obesity skyrocketed, the seventies looked like the good old days.

The slow but insistent growth of obesity as a health crisis received a huge catalyst in the 1990s, when two studies showed that obesity rates had increased steadily and dramatically during the 1980s and early 1990s. First to make news were the results of the third phase of the National Health and Nutrition Examination Survey (NHANES), performed between 1988 and 1994. The study found that obesity rates among American adults had increased to 22.5 percent from 14.5 percent in the late 1970s. Then, in 1999, the Centers for Disease Control (CDC) released the results of telephone surveys conducted between 1991 and 1998. In those eight years, they reported, the percentage of obese Americans increased by half; there were eleven million more obese people in 1998 than there had been in 1991.[34] Critics have argued that the reportedly dramatic rise in obesity rates during the 1990s may have been caused by statistical manipulation of a relatively small weight increase, and others point out that of the newly obese, twenty-nine million became so suddenly, when the National Institutes of Health released new weight guidelines in 1998.[35] Nonetheless, the data alarmed the public-health community and led to increasingly vigorous attempts, on federal, state, and local levels, to combat the trend.

Like other modern dietary-reform movements, the campaign that took shape in the mid- to late 1990s to combat obesity also redefined and expanded the purview of dietary reform. In the context of obesity, dietary advice cut a broader swath across the experiences and activities of daily life than ever before. This expansion across the realms of daily life was related to a shift in emphasis from an empirical accounting of dietary intake to the measurement of body size. Negative nutrition entailed a set of guidelines that carefully prescribed the amounts and kinds of nutrients people should consume. But the focus on obesity as the nation's primary dietary health crisis brought new scrutiny to the size and shape of individual bodies and extended the impact of dietary advice well beyond eating habits.

While nutrition science remained an important resource for obesity reformers, body size—rather than eating habits—became the primary empirical measure of dietary health. Investment in body size as a health factor, indicator, and determinant evolved over the course of the twentieth century through a gradual, complex social and medical process. The central calculative tool of the antiobesity campaign, the Body Mass Index (BMI), was designed in the 1830s to determine population averages based on the relationship between height and weight. The use of the height-to-weight relationship as a measure of population norms morphed into the assessment of health based on those same norms in the 1940s. The Metropolitan Life Insurance Company tracked the death rate relative to height-to-weight norms and published a table showing what they called "ideal weights," or the weight at which a person had the longest life span. By the 1950s, the MetLife tables had become widely accepted as the authoritative determinant of who was overweight. Once the tables were adopted by doctors, epidemiologists, and the federal government to analyze the health of the population, body size became a cultural repository for the idea of health. Though the BMI was established as a way to predict early death, the use of height-to-weight tables caused people to believe that body fat was in fact the cause of early death.[36] Since diet was at the same time becoming central to a new culture of health that emphasized the relationship between chronic diseases and lifestyle, and since eating habits were believed to be directly linked to body size, the BMI gradually became an authoritative measure of "eating right."[37]

Once body size became emblematic of health, a whole range of activities beyond eating habits was drawn into the realm of dietary reform, expanding dramatically its cultural purview and significance. Obesity was far more central to health concerns overall than earlier dietary crises had been, in an era in which health concerns were far more central to the culture overall than they had previously been. Consequently, claims of expertise over the new dietary crisis arose from myriad professions. Nutritional science, with its focus on the physiological relationship between food intake and health, was but one of many logics laying claim to the problem. Frameworks for understanding and addressing the problem of obesity also arose from the realms of genetics, psychology, exercise physiology, urban planning, and social-justice activism, among others. Exercise and eating habits remained the primary (though contested) focus of the debate over etiology, but theories about genetic underpinnings and social causes also became widely accepted (though contested).[38] Alongside significant debates about the details, by the early twenty-first century there was general agreement among popular and professional opinions that population weight gain had been caused by changes in the physical and social environment in the second half of the twentieth century that made nutrient-dense food more accessible and physical activity less so.

Despite this generally accepted framework for understanding the rise in weight, debate about the precise causes and appropriate treatments for obesity continued. The conversation about the possible causes of obesity also extended the purview of dietary reform by casting suspicion on almost every aspect of daily life. Much of the focus was on factors related to diet and exercise (fast food, increasing portion sizes, high fructose corn syrup, elevators, television, video games, urban design that discouraged walking). But these possible causes were also joined by an extensive array of factors not directly related to diet or exercise (air conditioning and heating, sleep deprivation, quitting smoking, popular medications, and older women giving birth).[39] As one satirical newspaper article explained, mutually contradictory reports about the causes of obesity included "your pop" (each serving of carbonated beverages consumed by a child increases risk of obesity by 60 percent), "your mom" (fetal exposure to sugar may alter the body's chemistry), genes, television, religion (religious people tend to weigh more), hormones, diet, and dieting (teenage girls who dieted and exercised with the intention of losing weight were found to be more likely to end up obese).[40] With so many aspects of daily life cast as possible causes of the obesity crisis, dietary reform was no longer a matter of teaching people how to eat right. Eating habits remained at the heart of the antiobesity campaign, but eating right was now considered inseparable from the extensive range of activities that were also considered related to weight gain.

As the empirical aspects of dietary reform shifted from calculating nutrient intake to measuring body size, so too did its moral aspects. The body became the visible sign of the same notions of morality and responsibility that other dietary-reform movements had invested in eating habits or the process of learning to eat right. The moral valence of body size within the antiobesity campaign drew on a long history of the symbolic association of fatness with moral weakness and flawed character. According to Amy Farrell, fatness was taken as a sign of inferiority and "out of control impulses" beginning in the nineteenth century, and cultural associations between fatness and primitiveness established at the brink of modernity remain with us today. Fatness was an important category within nineteenth- and early-twentieth-century thinking on evolution, an attribute seen as "demarcating the divide between civilization and primitive culture, whiteness and blackness, good and bad."[41] At the same time, as Peter Stearns points out, weight control became a "moral compensation" that allowed middle-class Americans to indulge in consumerism while retaining their commitment to personal restraint through the exercise of discipline over the body.[42] Increased affluence and consumerism after World War II led to an intensification of the ethical imperative to diet, and the thin body became "a sign of an ability to resist temptation and unwanted appetite, a guarantor of moral reliability."[43] This took place within a growing cultural investment in the visual assessment of bodies that also occurred in the second half of the twentieth century, causing the shape and size of bodies to be increasingly taken as a sign of character and morality.[44]

The reorientation of the culture of health around chronic diseases heightened the existing social significance of body size by refocusing the discourse and strategies of public health around the behavior and appearance of bodies. By the late 1960s, health problems were increasingly understood as within individual control, the terrain of activities considered linked to health had expanded significantly, and the pursuit of health had become an increasingly important aspect of people's everyday lives, their sense of their own subjectivity and morality, and their assessment of others. As this new ideological formation, or "new health consciousness," swept Americans up in a moral and social imperative to pursue health, maintaining a healthy weight became the central health and moral problem in many people's lives. Speaking of the final decades of the twentieth century, Robert Crawford observes, "When people talk about health as a goal, they are often describing their desire to lose weight. To be healthy is to be thin, literally, to be 'in shape.'"[45]

The extent of the moral investment in the empirical measure of body size was particularly evident in the fact that many dieters were willing to compromise or sacrifice their health in order to achieve the ultimate sign of health—a thin body. Health was ostensibly the goal of the antiobesity movement and of individual weight-loss efforts, but studies showed that many people would be willing to forfeit health and longevity to attain thinness. One study found that 91 percent of 273 dieters surveyed would *not* take a pill that would increase their life expectancy if such a pill guaranteed that they would become and remain overweight.[46] A survey of overweight and obese patients conducted in 2004 at Harvard Medical School revealed that 19 percent of overweight and 33 percent of obese people were willing to risk death for even a modest 10 percent weight loss, and many were willing to give up some of the remaining years of their lives if they could live those years weighing only slightly less.[47] These studies may have reflected the fact that dieters were willing to die earlier to lose weight in order to live remaining years in healthier, more able bodies, but studies also showed that people were willing to trade obesity for serious physical impairments. According to one, five year olds would choose to lose an arm rather than become fat. Almost all formerly fat weight-loss surgery patients in another study agreed that they would rather lose a leg than be fat.[48] These striking findings show that thinness operated as a sign of physical health and moral fortitude independently of other measures of health, and they suggest exactly how compelling the moral valence of body size was becoming.

The investment in body size as a marker of health and morality was heightened by the framing of obesity as a dangerous epidemic. The use of the term *epidemic* to describe obesity grew in part out of a population-centered approach to dietary health, but it was also a strategy used to both express and generate emotional urgency. The transition to a public-health emphasis on chronic disease and the emergence of negative nutrition were accompanied by a shift toward health strategies aimed at population-level results. While the Basic 7 and other food-group approaches to dietary advice (such as the four food groups of the postwar era) addressed the food choices of individuals, the dietary guidelines of the late twentieth century were aimed at the average diet of citizens. They were designed to improve the diet of the population overall and to reduce the prevalence of certain diseases based on a national average. For example, the guidelines of negative nutrition, including those aimed at reducing obesity, were intended largely to reduce the prevalence of heart disease among the population. But since coronary risk was greatest among middle-aged men, the rest of the population may have achieved no individual benefit from following them. The mass-population approach to disease prevention sought to persuade everyone to change their habits in order to reduce risk factors in the whole population, even though relatively few people were likely to avoid disease by following the advice that was issued.[49]

Approaching health in terms of population averages rather than individual risks or benefits fostered a population-level discourse on obesity, one that imagined rising weight among individuals as a dangerous tide slowly but steadily engulfing the entire nation. The image of the national body being overtaken by the rising rate of obesity became just as iconic as the fat body itself, in large part due to a striking visual representation of statistical changes in individual body weight. In 1989 William Dietz, the director of the Division of Nutrition and Physical Activity at the CDC, produced the first—startling, captivating—visual representation of the nation endangered by obesity expressly to convince Americans that obesity represented an urgent threat not just to fat individuals but to the nation as a whole. He designed a set of maps of the United States that used different colors to show rising rates of overweight and obesity in each state (see figure 5.1). Abstracting the statistics to the level of state weight gains exacerbated alarm since red in New York registered the same as red in Kansas, for example, despite the difference in the number of individuals it represented.[50]

Moving from cool blues to alarming reds as obesity rose over time, the maps dramatically envisioned the increasing body mass of individual Americans as a danger spreading across the national land mass. Presented in a PowerPoint format, the maps animated a lifeless set of data, shocking audiences and convincing people that obesity was happening not just to individuals, but to the nation, and that it was spreading dangerously across the United States like a virus.[51] The slides, and the ideas about the nature of the obesity threat that they so powerfully visualized, also spread much like a virus. Once made available online, they were instantly and incessantly reproduced in presentations and publications to reinforce the perspective that obesity was happening to people, much like a disease, and that it was spreading rapidly, much like an epidemic. Dietz himself remarked that his visuals "shifted the discussion from whether or not a problem existed to what we should do about the epidemic."[52]

Antiobesity reformers and the media perpetuated the framing of obesity as an epidemic, upping the moral ante of dietary health despite the fact that obesity was clearly not an epidemic in the true sense of the word. As Saguy and Riley point out, the term originally referred to "the rapid and episodic onset of infectious diseases" and was "associated with fear and sudden widespread death." Today, they explain, the term *epidemic* has come to be used as an "emotionally charged metaphor," the intent of such usage—with regard to drug addiction, for example, as well as to obesity—being "to clothe certain undesirable yet blandly tolerated social phenomenon in the emotional urgency associated with a 'real' epidemic."[53] But the language of the obesity epidemic drew on both the literal and the meta-

FIGURE 5.1 • Body-mass increases steadily engulfing the national land mass from 1985 to 2010. Digital rendering of CDC slides.

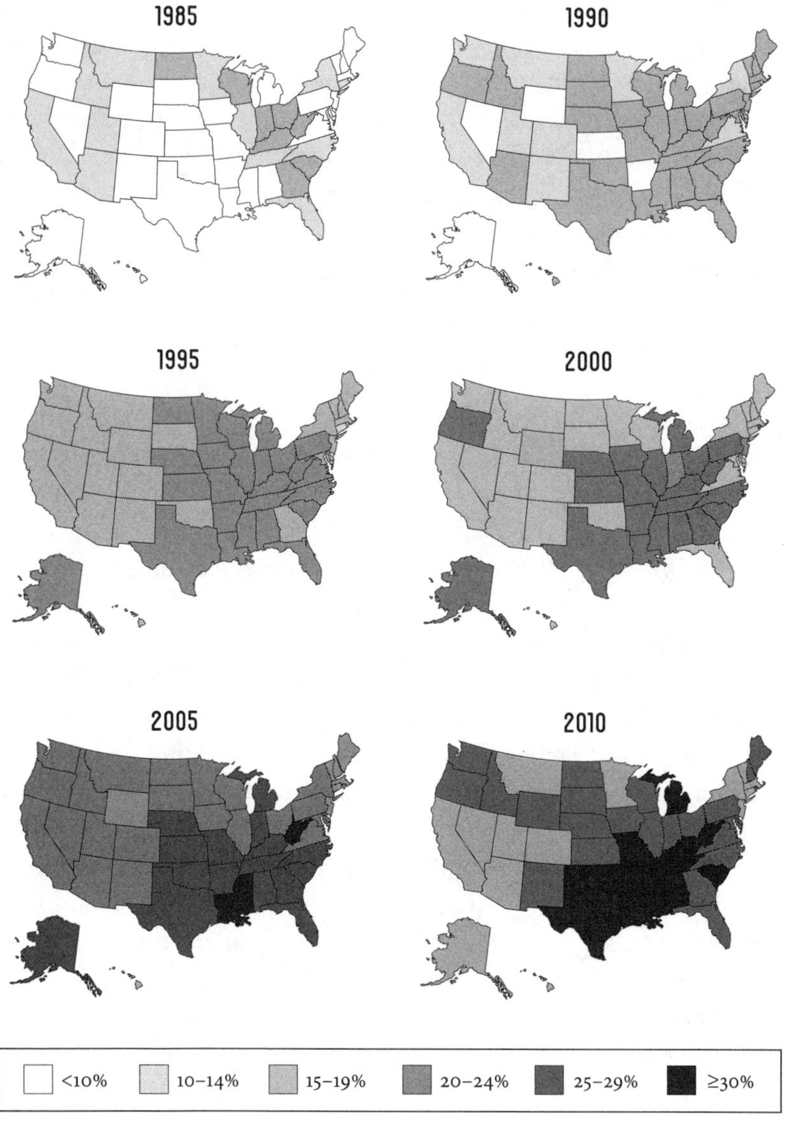

phoric implications of the term. Maps portraying obesity as a spreading infection, along with research arguing that obesity was "socially contagious," implied that obesity was a literal epidemic despite the fact that it was clearly not an infectious disease.[54]

The notion of obesity as a dangerous epidemic requiring an immediate response captured the historical changes in the culture of health, the prevailing nutritional paradigm, and the meaning of eating right that had occurred since World War II. Obesity had become a prevailing health concern and a pervasive moral symbol. The historical imperative to "eat right" had been transferred to body size and diffused across the realms of daily life. And the campaign against obesity was beginning to undertake the cultural work of dietary reform, adapting people to changes in the meaning of good citizenship.

Thinness, Self-Control, and Citizenship

By the late 1990s, a conversation about what "we should do about the epidemic" was raging. In 1994 there were about 33 news stories declaring obesity an epidemic. In 1995 the number of articles about obesity published in medical journals began to rise dramatically, and a spike in media reporting followed. By 2000, the number of stories regarding obesity was up to 107, and in 2004 there were nearly 700.[55]

In 2001, not long after the September 11 attacks on the Pentagon and the World Trade Center, the federal government launched its official "war against obesity" with the publication of *The Surgeon General's Call to Action to Prevent and Decrease Overweight and Obesity*. This pamphlet drew on the new visual language of obesity, opening with a pair of maps, under the heading "The Surfacing of an Epidemic," that depicted the prevalence of obesity among adults in 1991 and 2001. Each state was shaded to represent the percentage of obesity among adults in its population, with the higher levels drawn in darker shades. Side by side, the two maps presented a contrast in light and dark that evoked and expressed alarm about the nation's darkening future and established the urgent necessity of action.[56] The response to this perceived threat drew on the ever-present moral aspects of nutrition and the historical relationship between dietary and social ideals. Like other dietary-reform movements, the campaign against obesity provided lessons in eating right that were also lessons in good citizenship, adjusting the population to prevailing understandings of citizenship in two ways. Above all, the discourse of the antiobesity campaign promoted the importance of self-control. Advice circulated around an equivalence of thinness, health, and self-control that expressed and validated fundamental American beliefs in autonomy and individualism, but also responded to the growing emphasis on personal responsibility that attended neoliberalization. Though not an official wartime nutrition program, the campaign against obesity also helped adapt citizens to the exigencies of the War on Terror "home front."

The primary message of antiobesity reform was that people needed to attain and maintain body weights (or BMIS) in the ideal range established by federal guidelines. Implied in this message was that people needed to access and assert their will in order to overcome the threat that obesity posed to both their own bodies and the social body writ large. Dietary reformers have historically provided lessons in eating right that doubled as lessons in good citizenship: domestic science conveyed the importance of ceding liberty to the law, and the National Nutrition Program used the language of dietary advice to promote social ideals related to good home-front citizenship, such as alertness, courage, and cooperativeness. Despite ongoing debates about the probable causes and possible solutions of the epidemic, the campaign against obesity consistently reinforced the social value of self-control. It insisted on an irrefutable equivalence between thinness and self-control that extended to an equivalence between thinness and fitness for citizenship.

The obsession with self-control drew on fundamental American tenets of good citizenship, but also responded to the heightened mandate for self-discipline that attended neoliberalization. As Crawford explains, "Self-control, self-denial and will power are concepts that are fundamental to the western system of values," and they have become "as inseparable from modern individualism as they have from our notions of adulthood, even personhood."[57] But the importance of self-control as a marker of legitimate personhood—and therefore fitness for citizenship—intensified in the context of the political-economic reorientations around individual autonomy that took place in the late twentieth century. One effect of neoliberalization was to shift responsibility for minimizing health risks and their related costs from the state to individuals. Health was reconfigured as a responsibility rather than a right, and citizens were increasingly expected to make responsible choices as consumers, to adopt preventative practices, and to exercise self-discipline.[58] As Julie Guthman explains, the neoliberal subject "is expected to exercise choice and become responsible for his or her risks. In that way, neoliberalism also produces hyper-vigilance about control and self-discipline."[59] In its insistence on the importance of self-control, obesity discourse may have not only reflected the values of neoliberalization but also played a role in advancing and normalizing them.[60]

The equation of thinness with self-control and the related self-control directive were everywhere evident in obesity discourse. Especially striking were instances where the equivalence was taken to trump experience. The authors of a diet book targeted at African American women, for example, insisted, "If you weigh more than is healthy you are out of control, even if you feel that your life is in control." They went on to assert that although her finances, employment, and relationships may all be under control, "a sister who is truly in control of her life would never put herself in [the] position" of becoming overweight or obese.[61] Conversely, in 2001 an article in the *New Yorker* reported that people who had undergone bariatric surgery in order to achieve massive weight loss received self-control along with thin bodies. A woman who had had the surgery said that "she felt a profound and unfamiliar sense of willpower. She no longer *had* to eat anything. . . . She knew, intellectually, that the surgery was why she no longer ate as much as she used to, yet she felt as if she were choosing not to do it."[62]

The drumbeat of self-control, a constant in dieting advice, was also striking in the context of communal weight-loss efforts designed to emphasize the power of the collective. In 2005 the National Body Challenge brought 150,000 Americans together to lose weight, holding weigh-ins in malls and forming an Internet community to support and guide dieters. The program's central focus was using the collective to urge individuals to muster their own wills. Its motto, printed on every page in the food journal participants were supposed to write in every day, was "If you have the will, we have the way." A smaller-scale community weight-loss program popularized in the book *The Town that Lost a Ton* also focused on team effort, with weight-loss teams such as the Meltaway Mammas and Hips Hips Away competing for the greatest numbers of pounds lost. There, too, the willpower of each individual was considered the linchpin of the team effort. Participants were encouraged to post encouraging phrases in their homes such as "Your IQ is not nearly as important as your will" and "Willpower is a muscle, the more you use it the stronger it becomes."[63]

The self-control message was also pushed by federal antiobesity initiatives under George W. Bush. Consistent with the president's ideological leanings, and in particular his embrace of a "culture of personal responsibility," Bush's antiobesity strategy minimized the government's role in health promotion and hinged on individual agency and willpower. In 2003 the Bush administration launched an initiative called HealthierUS that both reflected and advanced a neoliberal reframing of health in which good citizens were expected to help control national health-care costs through practices of prevention and responsible consumption.[64] HealthierUS called on people to take responsibility for their own health and the well-being of the nation by being physically active every day, developing good eating habits, taking advantage of preventative screening, and making "healthy choices." In a speech launching the initiative, Bush celebrated the links between public-health reform and individual responsibility: "One of the things I talk a lot about is the need to really work on cultural change in America to encourage a culture of personal responsibility. . . . The HealthierUS initiative really appeals to personal responsibility, doesn't it? It says that we are responsible to our own health. . . . By making healthy choices we can do the right thing for our future." Bush explained that obesity both caused health problems and added to the cost of health care. Reinforcing the duty of citizens to minimize health-care costs, he remarked, "Good foods and regular exercise will reverse the trend, and save our country a lot of money—but, more importantly, save lives." Bush also argued that personal responsibility and self-control were the most important parts of his "preventative health care program": "We'll work on health care matters, we're working on Medicare reform. . . . But the truth of the matter is, one of the best reforms in America for health care is a strong, preventative health care program that starts with each American being responsible for what he or she eats . . . drinks . . . doesn't smoke . . . whether or not they get out and exercise." For those needing a little help with discipline, he advised using the online "self-policing mechanism" made available as part of the HealthierUS initiative.[65] This approach exemplified the process of "responsibilization," or imposing of responsibilities, that was integral to the production of neoliberal citizens.[66] The Obama administration followed with Let's Move, an antiobesity program that was decidedly more focused on structural changes. In addition to encouraging changes in individual behavior, it encouraged structural changes that would, for example, improve school lunches and make healthy foods more affordable and accessible. But like other "environmental" approaches to obesity, Let's Move ultimately reinforced the primacy of personal responsibility and self-control.

By the time Barack Obama took office, a growing body of scientific research and popular publications had led to an emerging consensus that the environment—that is, structural factors outside of individual control—played a significant role in weight gain. First introduced in the late 1990s as the "obesogenic environment" thesis, the theory focused on ways in which the environments in which most Americans lived fostered an imbalance between energy intake and energy expenditure—too much energy dense food and too little exercise and other activity.[67] In 2004 Kelly Brownell, director of the Yale Center for Eating and Weight Disorders, published *Food Fight*, which contributed to shifting public opinion with its forceful argument that willpower was no match for a "toxic environment" that made it easy to eat too much and exercise too little. "The choices people make are important," Brownell argued, "but the nation has played the willpower and restraint cards for years and finds itself trumped again and again by an environment that overwhelms the resources of most people."[68] He called for environmental interventions such as designing activity-friendly communities, curbing food marketing in public schools, requiring food labeling in restaurants, and changing the cost structure of food to make healthy foods less costly than unhealthy foods.[69] Michael Pollan also advanced the environmental approach to antiobesity reform with publications throughout the 2000s arguing that obesity was a result of agricultural policies that had caused the cost of calories to "plummet" since the 1970s.[70] "When food is abundant and cheap," Pollan argued in *The Omnivore's Dilemma* (2006), "people will eat more of it and get fat."[71] In his *In Defense of Food* (2008), Pollan explained that the industrialization of the American diet, the rise of highly processed foods, and "the superabundance of cheap calories of sugar and fat produced by modern agriculture" were to blame for obesity and other problems: "That such a diet makes people sick and fat we have known for a long time."[72]

Despite the increasing acknowledgment among antiobesity reformers and the general public that population weight gain was caused at least in part by factors outside of individual control, the idea that obesity represented a failure of self-discipline and thus marked fat people as failed citizens remained unshakeable. The intention of the toxic-environment thesis was to remove willpower and thus morality from the equation, but, as many critics have pointed out, it ultimately failed to do so. The theory did not, for example, account for how some people managed to become or remain thin within the same environment that caused others to become fat, leaving open the implication that willpower was still the critical determinant of thinness and health. As Guthman argues, whether the blame is put to productivist agriculture, an overly lax regulatory environment, food marketing run amok, or inadequacies in food accessibility, "When all is said and done the argument still places responsibility on the individual."[73]

While the idea that obesity was caused at least in part by environmental factors caught on among the public, the equivalence between body-size ideals (thinness) and prevailing social ideals (self-control) remained entrenched. Research showed that despite the fact that many Americans believed there were structural factors that caused obesity and acknowledged that weight loss was nearly impossible, they were nonetheless unwilling to let go of the primacy of personal responsibility and the imperative to self-control. A 2001 poll, for example, showed that many Americans already supported the idea that there were important environmental causes of obesity: 62 percent agreed that too much unhealthy food in restaurants and supermarkets was to blame, and 57 percent agreed that diets were ineffective. The same poll also showed, however, that most of those same people nonetheless remained convinced that fatness was ultimately due to a failure of self-control: 65 percent of respondents believed that lack of willpower was the main cause of obesity.[74] A 2009 study based on survey data from 456 people and in-depth interviews with 42 "overweight" respondents also showed that "moral models of fatness" remained pervasive despite growing acknowledgment of structural factors, particularly corporate culpability. The study found that many people placed responsibility on both individuals and corporations, but they "adamantly voiced that individuals have free will, make their own decisions, and therefore should not blame the food industry," and they insisted that "fat individuals are unrestrained and lack self-control." The most agreed-on point was that people could, and should, control their own body size. Of the respondents, 93.3 percent "felt that overweight or fat individuals are responsible for their own bodies. Only 1.5 percent expressed any form of dissent."[75] Self-identified "overweight" people in the study also understood their own experiences through this pervasive, moralizing frame. A thirty-four-year-old Hispanic man explained, for example, "'Well, I gained the weight because I ate. I wasn't active. Therefore to lose the weight, [I need to] watch what I eat, get active. You can control these things. These things are in your control.'"[76]

The equivalence between health, thinness, and self-control pervaded obesity discourse, functioning as a pedagogy of good citizenship for the early twenty-first century. Talking about weight and health reinforced the primacy of personal responsibility and the mandates for self-control and responsible consumption that were central to the political, economic, and social ethos of neoliberalism. But lessons in eating right in the context of obesity were shaped not only by the demands of neoliberalization, but also by the related pressures of post-9/11 political and social adjustments. The nation declared its war against obesity and its war against terror in the same two-month period. As the two campaigns took shape, they occasionally overlapped in obvious ways, but, perhaps less evidently, they also collaborated in the construction of a post-9/11 collective and a pervasive sense of endangerment that served important political purposes on the terror "home front." While clearly not an explicit wartime dietary-reform campaign in the same sense as World War II's National Nutrition Program, the campaign against obesity subtly took on the features of a wartime propaganda campaign, helping to sustain the social conditions conducive to the war effort and promoting eating right as a form of good wartime citizenship.[77]

The convergence of the discourses of obesity and terror began very soon after the 9/11 attacks, which coincided with a dramatic surge in media reporting about obesity.[78] A catastrophe of such scale could have eclipsed worries about how much Americans weighed, yet news stories on the latest research about growing waistlines were among the first not directly related to the attacks and their aftermath to appear in the fall of 2001.[79] In December 2001, just months after the 9/11 attacks, the government officially launched its antiobesity campaign with the publication of *The Surgeon General's Call to Action to Prevent and Decrease Overweight and Obesity* (dedicated to one of its senior editors, who died on September 11).[80] Around this same time, news reports began to reframe obesity as a threat to national security. In November 2001, for example, Reuters ran the headline "U.S. Male Soldiers Are Getting Fatter."[81] An article in the *Washington Times* declared half of the U.S. military overweight in January 2002, the same month that Bush delivered his State of the Union speech identifying Iraq as part of the "axis of evil" and vowing not to let dangerous regimes threaten the United States with destructive weapons.[82] The article directly positioned obesity as a potential threat to military aims: "Overweight troops can hinder not only their own performance but that of their units as well as the success of their often grueling military missions."[83]

Though simultaneous to and overlapping with concerns about obesity, the War on Terror did not turn the antiobesity campaign into an explicit defense issue as mobilization had for hidden hunger. The campaign against obesity was waged parallel to, instead of as part of the War on Terror, but it did fulfill some of the functions of a wartime morale campaign, helping to unite the nation in a common cause and against a shared enemy despite the fact that this war lacked a clearly defined target, had no definite goals, and was not supported by a draft or propaganda campaigns that explicitly channeled civilian energy into the national cause. Especially throughout the early years of the campaign, weight loss was frequently framed as a patriotic duty and a requirement of good wartime citizenship. At the December 2001 launch of the "national plan of action" in response to obesity, for example, Secretary of Health and Human Services Tommy G. Thompson explicitly positioned weight loss as a duty to the nation when he declared, "All Americans should lose 10 pounds as a patriotic gesture."[84] Federal officials frequently reinforced this framing of weight loss as a patriotic act: President Bush was reported to have asked White House staff members on a daily basis whether they had done their workouts, and Thompson himself publicly shed fifteen pounds and wore a pedometer to work every day.[85] Media representations of the antiobesity campaign added to the patriotic aura of weight loss through the use of evocative iconography. Images of a fat Uncle Sam appeared frequently to express the threat that obesity posed to the nation and national identity. A 2004 *Harvard Magazine* cover used the image of a fat, flag-draped lady liberty to convey the connection between the obesity epidemic and national character (see figure 5.2). It evoked a distant memory of a better past and a sense of national shame by depicting the flag-draped lady liberty standing on a penny scale, aghast at the display, yet holding a cornucopia overflowing with beer cans, soda bottles, peanut butter, and chips instead of the wholesome, iconic foods of the American harvest.[86] Years later, after the urgency of the War on Terror had waned, the patriotic iconography of obesity remained salient. Strikingly, a 2010

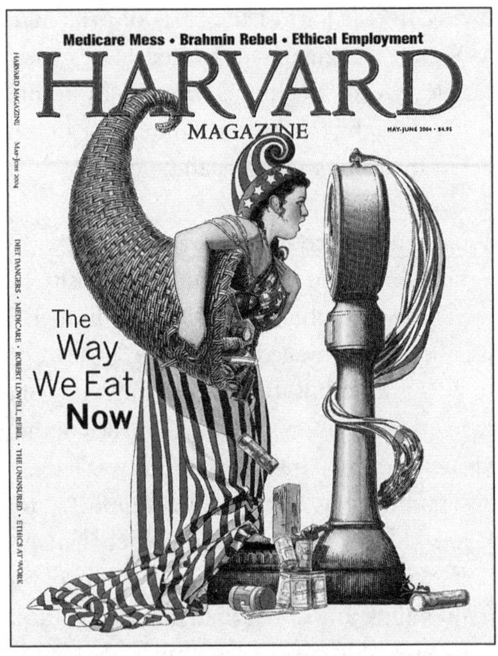

FIGURE 5.2 • Patriotic iconography of obesity. Cover of *Harvard Magazine*, May–June 2004.

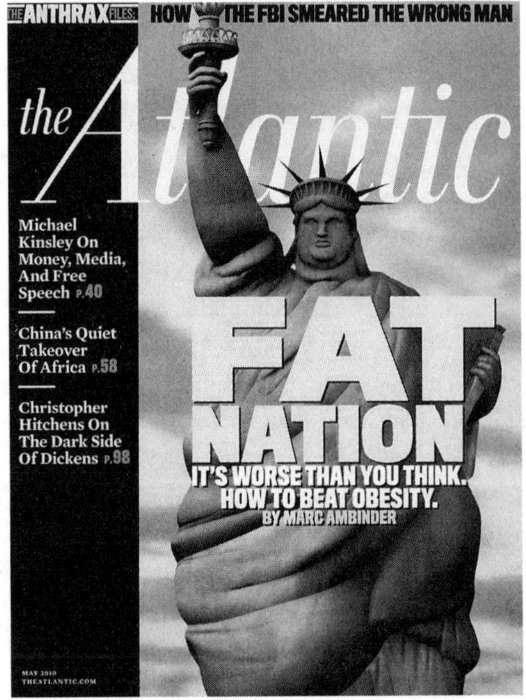

FIGURE 5.3 • Patriotic iconography of obesity. Cover of the *Atlantic*, May 2010.

cover for the *Atlantic* reprised both the anthrax story of the early years of the War on Terror and, through its depiction of a fat Statue of Liberty, the idea that obesity, like terrorism, threatened the essence of American identity and values (see figure 5.3).

The campaign against obesity provided civilians on the home front a set of seemingly achievable goals and a sense of communal purpose that the War on Terror lacked. In 2003 Surgeon General Richard Carmona, who was appointed by President Bush six months after 9/11, began delivering a series of speeches that both fueled fears about the threat of obesity and celebrated the fact that the problem of obesity had a clear and accessible solution. In these speeches, Carmona repeatedly referred to obesity as "the terror within." Explaining this in an interview on National Public Radio, Carmona remarked, "I've come to refer to it as the terror within because it's every bit as devastating as terrorism."[87] He called obesity "a threat that is every bit as real to America as the weapons of mass destruction."[88] While he portrayed obesity and terror as equally menacing threats lurking within national borders, Carmona suggested that the war against obesity was easily winnable through the dedicated efforts of citizens working toward a common purpose. "The good news," he announced, "is that this health crisis is almost entirely preventable through proper diet and exercise." While the War on Terror was characterized by its elusive enemy, poorly defined aims, and seemingly endless nature, Carmona dispensed a "simple prescription that [could] end America's obesity epidemic: every American needs to eat healthy food in healthy portions and be physically active every day."[89] Carmona's pronouncements reinforced neoliberal responsibilization while also making collective efforts toward weight loss a meaningful way for individuals to practice good wartime citizenship by participating in a national struggle against a mortal threat.

By urging Americans to eat less, make healthier choices, and exercise more, the war against obesity provided the focus for communal effort and self-sacrifice that the War on Terror lacked. While there were immediate calls for Americans to give blood and money in the wake of the 9/11 attacks, the War on Terror notably lacked a campaign for material sacrifice among citizens. On the contrary, government and industry leaders urged Americans to keep spending and buying in order to "Keep America Rolling," as General Motors put it.[90] At the same time, however, the war against obesity called for extreme sacrifice and self-denial. Americans were exhorted to give up their favorite foods, eat less, and exercise every day. President Bush's ambitious goal of getting "20 million additional Americans to exercise for at least 30 minutes a day, five days a week" exemplified the displacement of calls for wartime sacrifice from the War on Terror to the war against obesity.[91]

The war against obesity, running parallel to that on terror, also helped to adapt the population to serious but subtle transformations in the social and political context. By exacerbating the overwhelming sense of fear that permeated post-9/11 life in the United States, the discourse of obesity helped to justify and legitimize the vaguely defined, resource-intensive, and socially intrusive War on Terror. While fear was a completely logical response to the terror attacks, it was also, as David Altheide argues, a strategy that the government used to ensure support for wartime political and social adjustments.[92] Obesity participated in the construction of a "politics of fear," which Altheide describes as "decision makers' promotion and use of audience beliefs and assumptions about danger, risk and fear in order to achieve certain goals."[93] The goals of the post-9/11 politics of fear included "widespread support for military expenditures and the public's tacit approval of civil liberty restrictions."[94] The prior construction of obesity not just as a health problem for individuals but also as an urgent threat to the nation itself added to its traction within the post-9/11 politics of fear. As Saguy and Riley point out, "Declaring an epidemic has historically lent a sense of urgency that can—like declaring war—justify abridging civil liberties."[95]

Alongside news reports and color-coded threat warnings suggesting the imminence of another terrorist attack, alarming reports about obesity exacerbated an overall sense of danger and unease. According to U.S. Surgeon General Richard Carmona, for example, "300,000 Americans a year die from [obesity's] complications, nearly 1,000 every day, one every 90 seconds. Obesity is an epidemic now, and it's growing. If we don't do anything about it, we will have a morbidly obese dysfunctional population that we cannot afford to care for."[96] While the "fact" that obesity was killing 300,000 Americans each year was the subject of ongoing controversy and debate, major news outlets repeated the alarming statistic over 17,000 times between 2002 and 2004.[97] The threat of obesity also exacerbated the post-9/11 sense that danger was everywhere. While the fear of impending terror attacks turned backpacks, garbage cans, delivery trucks, and running water into potential weapons, the war against obesity located deadly threats in grocery stores and on dinner plates. Potential causes for the deadly epidemic propagated by research studies and media reports included everything from snacking to sodas and air conditioning. In a 2003 speech the U.S. surgeon general listed computers, television, elevators, close parking spots, fast food, and microwave dinners among the aspects of everyday life that imperiled the health of the nation.[98] In a 2002 op-ed piece, a critic of the War on Terror described a terrifying landscape of deadly threats in the average American supermarket aisle: "We could use some weapons inspectors right here in our supermarkets. Who needs nerve gas when we have stockpiles of sugar, salt, and fat slowly immobilizing our children?" He continued, "Body fat is every bit as much a bioterrorist threat as anything Saddam might lob over."[99] Together, the everyday dangers posed by obesity and terror established a pervasive sense of fear that may have helped induce the population to accept wartime social changes, such as granting more power to political leaders and accepting new restrictions on civil liberties in exchange for protection and security.[100]

While the antiobesity campaign had absolutely no official connection to the War on Terror, a popular diet program provides a striking example of how the campaign against obesity nonetheless functioned as a wartime propaganda campaign by both enhancing the culture of fear and providing lessons in good wartime citizenship. The 2004 National Body Challenge was among the many communal weight-loss efforts that involved Americans in managing their dietary health for the good of the nation. A nationwide diet sponsored by the Discovery Health Network, the National Body Challenge provided 150,000 dieters online instruction and support. A companion television series involved viewers in the drama of six "body challengers" chosen to represent the nation and its struggle to lose weight (see figure 5.4). The first episode of *The National Body Challenge*, "The Battle Begins," which aired in the winter of 2003–2004, clearly situated obesity as a threat to national security. It began with shots of the challengers dressed in red, white, and blue in front of the United States Capitol while a narrator announced that the battle against obesity would begin at "one of the world's toughest military training grounds, just outside the nation's capital": the marine training base in Quantico, Virginia (see figure 5.5). The six challengers arrived at the marine base dressed in fatigues and ran through a series of strenuous, muddy obstacles in freezing temperatures (see figure 5.6). Slow-motion images of the fat Americans wheezing, crawling, crying, and collapsing as they struggled to com-

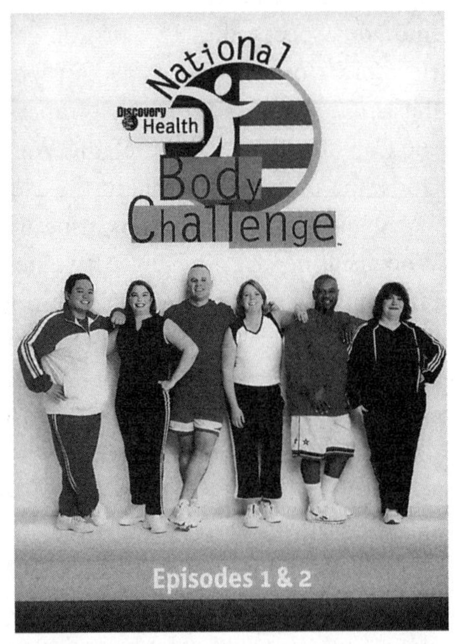

FIGURE 5.4 • *Right.* The *National Body Challenge* DVD cover. *National Body Challenge*, Discovery Health Channel (2004).

FIGURE 5.5 • *Below.* The body challengers in front of the Capitol building. Still from *National Body Challenge*, Discovery Health Channel (2004).

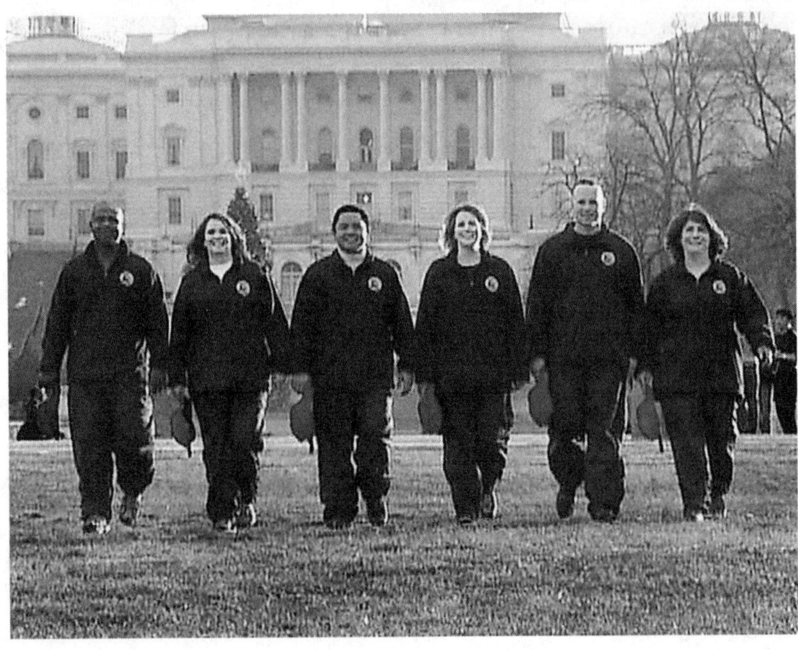

plete the course became the motivating backdrop for the rest of the series, with key parts—such as an ambulance rushing "the most defeated of them all" away from the course—replayed in every episode that followed.

Together with scenes in subsequent episodes of overweight firefighters struggling to run up stairwells and fat nurses barely able to transport stretchers through hospital hallways, these images portrayed obesity as a threat to the nation's ability to defend itself and respond to future attacks. Weight loss, in this context, was a patriotic wartime imperative. Celebrated as the focal point for a nationwide communal effort, the challengers participated in public weigh-ins, where each stepped onto a massive scale in front of cheering crowds in iconic communal settings throughout the country, such as midcourt at a Chicago Bulls game and at a Six Flags amusement park in Atlanta. Before-and-after photo shoots, in which contestants wore red-and-blue workout clothes and posed in front of red-and-white-striped backdrop, drew attention to their personal transformations as patriotic contributions to two simultaneous national wars. And those "body challengers," of course, were at the same time icons of good neoliberal citizenship, proudly taking on the responsibility to pursue and attain health through careful choices and self-discipline (see figure 5.7).

The Healthy Self and the Fat Other

Eating right in the era of obesity, as always, was both a duty equated with good citizenship and an identity that located individuals within the social hierarchy. But the social stakes were extremely high, higher than they had been in the context of any other modern dietary-reform movement. Fatness was a more visible stigma than bad eating habits, and most people believed that a fat body was evidence of a failure of self-control. Body size was also considered an incontrovertible sign of health or illness, and health was more central to identity and social status than it had been in other eras of dietary reform. The epidemic frame also contributed to the high social stakes for eating right, upping the emotional ante by casting obesity as a rapidly spreading, vaguely contagious threat to the nation as a whole. The social stigma related to obesity was also exacerbated by the hypervigilance around self-discipline that attended neoliberalization. Because individual responsibility had become such an important aspect of health and good citizenship, bad health was more than ever considered a personal failure that indicated a lack of the kind of autonomy and self-regulation required

KAREN

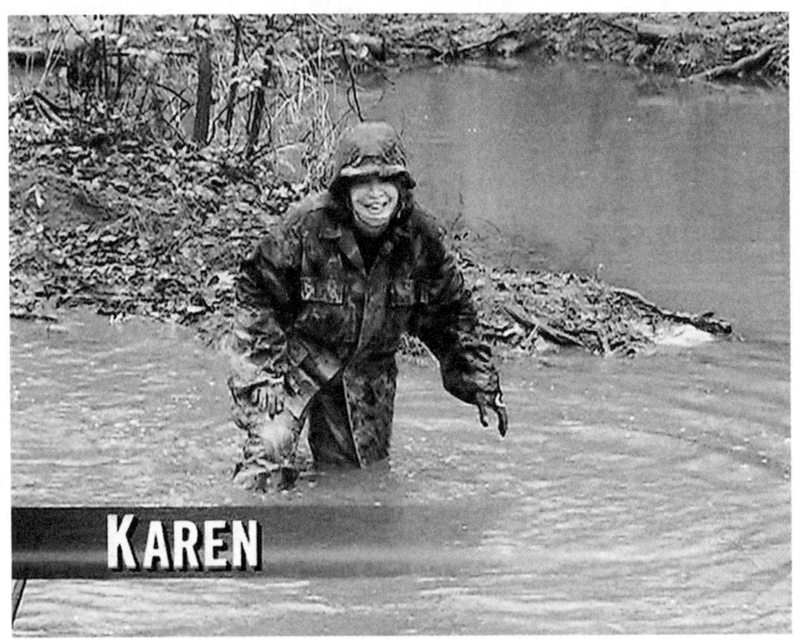

FIGURE 5.6 • A body challenger struggles to complete a marine training course. Still from *National Body Challenge*, Discovery Health Channel (2004).

Weight 219
Target 165
Body Fat 34.7%
Target 22.0%

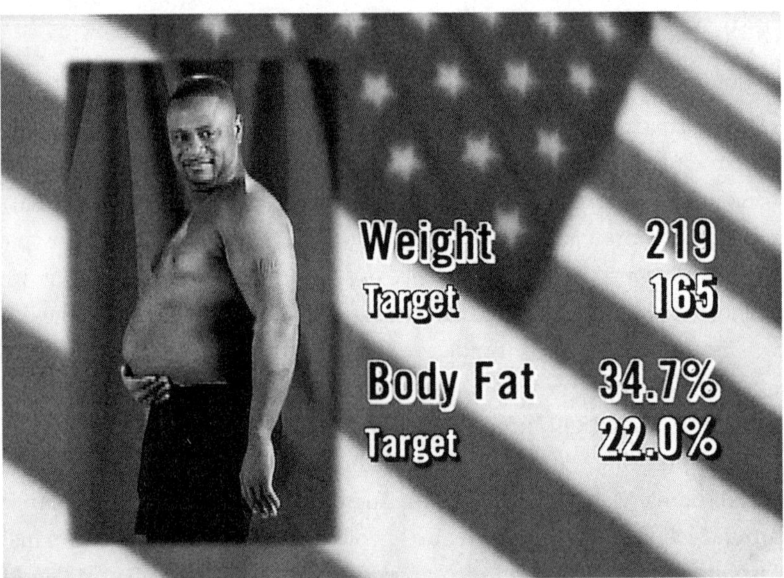

FIGURE 5.7 • A body challenger and his self-improvement targets framed by the American flag. Still from *National Body Challenge*, Discovery Health Channel (2004).

for good citizenship.[101] This stigma was directed at fat people, who suffered on a day-to-day basis from severe forms of prejudice and discrimination. The stigma of obesity also colluded virulently with existing race and class prejudice. Like earlier dietary-reform movements, the war against obesity bolstered (upper-)middle-class identity by identifying people of color and the poor with bad eating habits and poor health.

As Michelle Obama stood in the White House Garden in 2009 explaining the importance of eating right, she noted that alarming rates of overweight and obesity among American children "climb even higher" in "Hispanic and African American communities" and declared the numbers "unacceptable."[102] But the belief that Hispanics, blacks, and the poor were more likely to be overweight or obese was not a new one, nor was it incidental. The notion that obesity was largely a problem of minorities and those with low socioeconomic status (SES) was integral to its emergence as a medical and social problem in the 1960s and 1970s. *Obesity and Health*, a 1966 review of available information on obesity noted that "Negro women tended to be heavier in all age groups than white women of corresponding heights" and that "there [was] less overweight among high socio-economic class, particularly among women."[103] The final report of the 1969 White House Conference on Food, Nutrition and Health pointed out that greater levels of overweight were found among "Negroes" and the poor.[104] In its recommendations for avoiding overweight, the 1977 *Dietary Goals for the United States* noted, "For unknown reasons, in the United States, this type of malnutrition is a more common burden among the poor than among the more wealthy."[105] When the obesity epidemic was officially declared around the turn of the millennium, these disparities remained a focal point. *The Surgeon General's Call to Action to Prevent and Decrease Overweight and Obesity*, which launched the government's campaign against obesity in 2001, presented data on the distribution of overweight by race, ethnicity, gender, age, and socioeconomic status that was subsequently cited widely in the scientific, medical, and popular press. As in the earlier findings, the greatest racial, ethnic, and SES discrepancies were found among women: "In general, the prevalence of overweight and obesity is higher in women who are members of racial and ethnic minority populations than in non-Hispanic white women." Among men, Mexican Americans tended to have a high prevalence of overweight and obesity, but the prevalence among non-Hispanic whites was slightly higher than among blacks.[106] Regarding the impact of SES on overweight and obesity, the report concluded, "For all racial and ethnic groups combined, women of lower socioeconomic status . . . are approximately fifty percent more likely to be obese than those with higher socioeconomic status."[107]

The construction of obesity as a health crisis may have in fact hinged on its historical association with people of color and the poor. The authors of a 1998 article in the *New England Journal of Medicine* suspected as much. Explaining that the evidence of obesity risks and weight-loss benefits were much less clear than reporting would suggest, the authors surmised that a reason "for the medical campaign against obesity may have to do with the tendency to medicalize behavior we do not approve of."[108] Furthermore, as Farrell argues, since the late nineteenth century fatness had been seen as a mark of inferiority, with fat people being placed low on the scale of civilization along with "natives," immigrants, criminals, and women. At the end of the twenty-first century, she writes, the fat body continued to function as "shorthand" for the uncivilized body, with particular salience where stigmas of race, sex, and class were also at play: "A fat body can threaten to unravel all the best efforts at upward mobility, conjuring up historical and cultural memories of that Great Chain of Being in which fatness was considered to be characteristic of the most primitive, most 'ethnic,' the most sexually loose females, the most *inferior* people." The obsession with Barack and Michelle Obama's slimness and fitness routines attests to the ways a thin body, by contrast, can be used to contest other stigmas related to inferiority and primitivism, such as race.[109]

The association of fatness with failure of self-control heightened its potency as a social stigma at this intersection of race, class, and body size. In the context of the revamped mandate for self-control in the late twentieth century, not only were the unhealthy perceived as lacking in self-control, but those who were perceived as lacking self-control—such as minorities and the poor—were "also perceived as diseased or as agents of disease."[110] Crawford argues that the late twentieth century also saw an increased obsession with protecting the boundaries of legitimate selfhood and, therefore, a greater investment in constructing "unhealthy others" against whom the dominant group could affirm its own identity. The result, he claims, was the development of "a fear, fascination, and sense of horror of the other—a non-self who is believed to assume all of the characteristics antithetical to conventional self-hood."[111] Obesity discourse circulated around exactly this fear, fascination, and sense of horror of a raced, classed "other" presumed to be "uncivilized" and lacking in qualities fundamental to personhood.

Despite their differences, and their intentions, a variety of theories seeking to explain minority obesity fed into the stigma at the intersection of race, class, and body size. Environmental theories that attempted to shift blame from individuals to structural factors, for example, transferred stigma from individuals to the values and behaviors of entire social groups. Theories that posited minorities as more likely to be obese than the rest of the population because they were culturally inclined toward high-calorie cuisines and low levels of physical activity simply shifted blame from personal to cultural failures.[112] So, too, did theories that female body ideals among blacks and Latinos contributed to obesity in those communities by encouraging full, round figures. For example, the *New York Times* reported on a study showing that aesthetic preferences among African Americans contributed to their obesity rates by normalizing body shapes that correlated to BMIs close to the "obese" range. Not surprisingly, the study found that white body ideals were congruent with medical norms. While white women began expressing dissatisfaction with their bodies at a BMI of 25, which was the starting point of the overweight category, black and Hispanic women did not express such dismay until they reached a BMI of 30, which was on the border of the official obese category.[113] Reflecting and reinforcing these findings, the authors of *Slim Down Sister*, a weight-loss guide for African American women, argued that high regard for larger bodies within black culture posed a danger to women's health. White women, they wrote, "are more apt to place health concerns first when it comes to food. . . . The bottom line is we simply are not as preoccupied with dieting as white women." Although high self-esteem among black women may be a good thing, they worried that "it is in many ways, a drawback that can compromise our future health."[114]

Environmental theories accounting for the prevalence of obesity among minorities also exacerbated existing prejudice because they tended to reinforce the equivalence between thinness and self-control. Even researchers who recognized structural causes frequently ended up holding individuals responsible and blaming minorities for their own misfortune. Saguy and Riley cite an interview with an antiobesity researcher who, in discussing why poor minority women were more likely to be heavy, explained, "Some woman who's living in the housing projects and has no husband and is trying to take care of four kids and is now off welfare and has to work and has all kinds of problems: for her, diet is not [a priority]. . . . I don't think they're really connected to the idea that they need to lose twenty-five pounds, and so they don't try it."[115] Saguy and Riley found that with regard to managing obesity, researchers who recognized structural causal factors frequently resorted to a "risky behavior frame" that imputed individual responsibility and implied that people had a "medical and moral responsibility to manage their weight."[116]

The belief that body size was something individuals could control if they only tried exacerbated the social stigma related to obesity and fueled the dangerous collusion between antifat and other forms of social bias. Many observers have noted that adherence to the ideology of individualism increased prejudice against both fat people and minorities.[117] Studies bearing out these connections included a 2001 comparison of the structures of prejudice against fat people in six nations. Researchers found that negative attitudes toward fatness were linked to beliefs about its controllability and that these effects were more pronounced in individualist cultures.[118] Research also showed that belief in the primacy of self-control was linked to coexisting negative attitudes toward fat people, minorities, and the poor. One study found that more than 80 percent of people who believed that blacks are "welfare dependent" or that the poor are "irresponsible" also believed that "overweight people are fat because they lack self-control." This figure was much higher than among the general population.[119] Another study concluded, "Negative attitudes towards the obese are highly correlated with negative attitudes towards minorities and the poor, such as the belief that all these groups are lazy and lack self-control and will power." Media reports on obesity that mentioned blacks, Latinos, or the poor were also found to be more likely to blame obesity on bad food choices and sedentary lifestyles than were reports that did not mention those social groups.[120]

Biological explanations for obesity among blacks and immigrants, although they eliminated the issue of controllability, also lent themselves to amplifying existing prejudice. In the context of the campaign against obesity, inherited biological differences that may have caused larger body size were recast as deficiencies that threatened the health of individuals and the well-being of the nation as a whole. The authors of *Slim Down Sister*, for example, argued that African American women needed their own weight-loss program because they were biologically and culturally different from other women: "When it comes to weight loss, sisters are different. Our bodies work differently; our minds and spirits need different motivations."[121] But the authors described black women's lower basal metabolism as a "biological disadvantage" that caused "obese sisters" to burn fewer calories a day at rest than white women.[122] Researchers also pointed to biological differences—or "disadvantages"—responsible for high levels of obesity among immigrants. The "thrifty gene" theory, articulated as early as 1962, posited that periods of feast and famine in the days of "our hunter-gatherer ancestors" left humans with a genetic predisposition to hoard fat in preparation for the next famine.[123] While people removed for several generations from the experience of starvation no longer responded to abundance by storing fat, studies argued, high rates of obesity among Native Americans and immigrants from other "food deprived cultures" may have been the result of the thrifty gene. For example, a 1997 study of Mayan immigrants from Guatemala living in Florida and Los Angeles proposed that large weight gains among immigrants were caused by "metabolic inheritance"; due to the history of cultural and political oppression and economic exploitation in Guatemala, the study argued, Mayan children were born with a "metabolic inclination to hold on to fat" and "[were] not equipped with the metabolic machinery to handle overeating" in the context of abundance.[124] The thrifty-gene theory not only recast difference as disadvantage, but also implied that recent immigrants were driven by "primitive" biological responses that made them particularly maladapted to the American environment.

Biological explanations for the high prevalence of obesity among minorities also helped to bolster the increasingly controversial ideological position that race and ethnicity were biological categories rather than cultural ones.[125] Theories that high obesity rates among blacks and immigrants were the result of biological differences blatantly challenged the increasingly prevalent notion that race and ethnicity were cultural constructions and provided visual "proof" in the form of fat bodies that such differences emerged from distinctions on the cellular level.[126] Biological theories of poor and minority obesity validated and stigmatized bodily difference. Fat-acceptance researcher Paul Campos refused to accept either set of claims, arguing, "The most crucial parallel between obesity and race in America is that both concepts are, at the most fundamental biological and medical levels, fictions." The effects of their collusion were nonetheless real. Campos writes, "Race and obesity both illustrate how the social effects of an idea can be very real, even if the idea that produces those effects happens to be false."[127]

Coupled with the sense that obesity was an out-of-control epidemic, biological arguments led to concerns about "the future of the race" reminiscent of those that motivated domestic science. For example, Greg Critser, author of *Fat Land*, worried that obesity threatened to multiply as fat immigrants produced fat children. The obesity rate among Mexican American children, he explained, bore this out: by fourth grade 32.4 percent of Mexican American girls and 43.4 percent of Mexican American boys were obese. Critser argued that fat parents influenced the fatness of their children through both the environment and genetics. He also cited a study showing that increases in obesity rates in the population may have been caused in part by the stigma of obesity causing fat people to mate with each other. This "assortive mating" led to more obesity in the population both by producing familial environments that created fat kids and by "accelerating the genetic expression of obesity." Recognizing that there "glimmers just a touch of the old eugenicist impulse" in these remarks, he argued that "recognizing such a reality might help prevent a eugenic reality." However parents became obese, he explained, it was indisputable that "fat parents are more likely—much more likely—to raise fat children, who are in turn more likely to be fat adults, who are then more likely to continue the daisy chain until . . . all Americans are overweight and obese."[128]

The association between obesity and minorities and the collusion of race, class, and body-size prejudice made the specter of obesity especially threatening for the "healthy self" whose social status depended on maintaining a thin body. Consistent with Crawford's argument that since the mid-1970s middle-class identity has been particularly invested in the boundary-maintaining work of delineating the healthy self from the sick or at-risk other, a survey of attitudes toward fat people found that middle-class whites experienced the strongest antifat sentiments.[129] But one did not need to conduct a survey to see that the affluent upper middle class was terrified of becoming fat and was aware of its social implications, which threatened both race and class status. Fatness remained a marker of inferiority that threatened to strip members of the white, affluent middle class of their class and race privilege.[130]

That the possibility of becoming fat threatened the social status of the "healthy" upper middle class was dramatically illustrated in all manner of popular culture, especially the many "fat suit" films that explored the social ramifications of body size. Eddie Murphy's *The Nutty Professor* was among the first of what would become a rash of fat-suit films, and though it appeared early in the obesity crisis (1996), it provided an especially vivid exploration of how changing body size threatened class identity (while also proving that the social threat of obesity pre-dated the "epidemic").[131] In the film Murphy plays Sherman Klump, a fat, insecure scientist desperate to lose weight who discovers a DNA-altering formula that transforms him for brief periods into Buddy Love, a slender womanizer, also played by Murphy, who is of entirely different habitus[132] (see figures 5.8 and 5.9). Though clearly a professional, the film frames Klump as lower middle class through scenes of meals with his extended family. In one scene Klump's father is dressed in overalls, there is bawdy behavior during dinner (sexual remarks from Granny and a fart contest that ends with Papa Klump "messing himself" at the table), and Papa Klump refuses to "take the damn garbage" out because he is busy watching *Roseanne*. In contrast, Love is depicted as clearly upper class; he wears fancy suits, speeds through town in a flashy red sports car, and consumes the foods of the elite. On his first date with the beautiful Ms. Purty (the romantic interest of both Love and Klump), Buddy Love, who shares Klump's appetite, consumes six T-bone steaks, five baked potatoes, and two servings of creamed spinach in an upscale comedy club (see figure 5.10). The class symbolism of this meal is in clear contrast to that of the meal Ms. Purty experiences on her date with the fat professor, who takes her home to eat with his family; there, the meal includes fried chicken, ribs, corn muffins, and sweet potatoes (with a side of farts) (see figure 5.11).[133] Because body size is understood as a physical marker connected to class, the DNA-altering formula transforms both the professor's body and his social status. The film was a reminder of the threat that obesity posed to the identity of the upper middle class. Because the dramatic bodily and identity changes were attributed to a "DNA-altering formula," the story also suggested that weight and class were not only directly related but also genetically determined, though potentially, and dangerously, malleable.

The cumulative effect of these many collusions between race, class, and body-size bias was discrimination against fat people. The "bad eater" accrued negatively valued social qualities in each of the prior dietary-reform movements, but never were the social ramifications as severe. Because bodies, rather than eating habits, carried the social freight of dietary health;

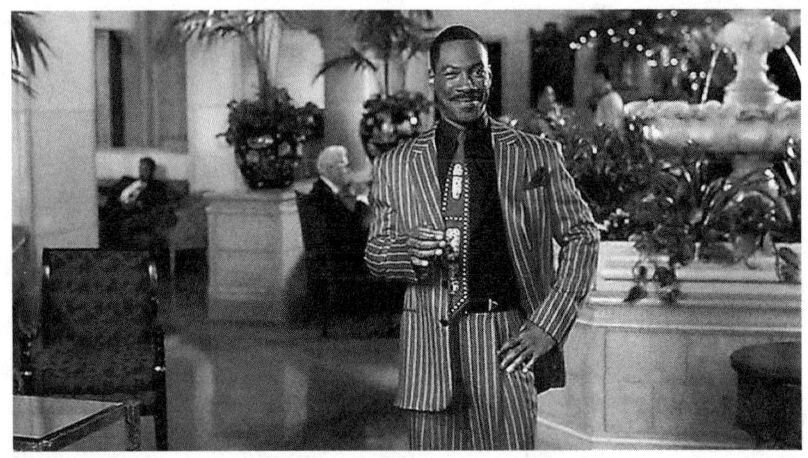

FIGURE 5.8 • Buddy Love. Still from *The Nutty Professor* (1996).

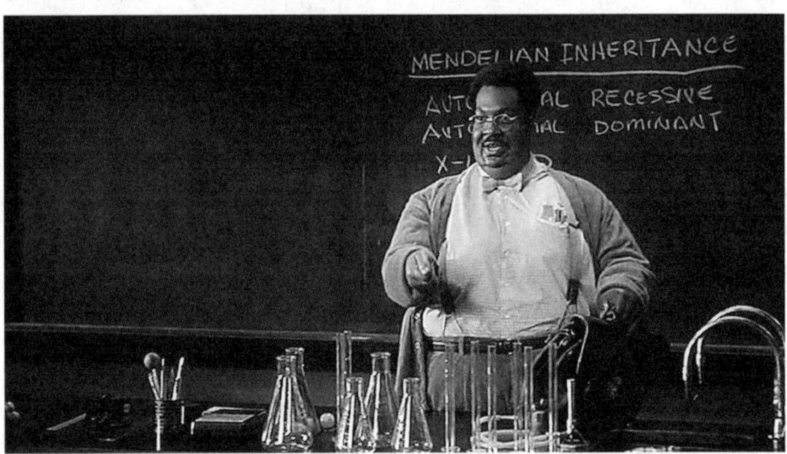

FIGURE 5.9 • Professor Klump. Still from *The Nutty Professor* (1996).

because the reform discourse so far exceeded the bounds of eating habits; because the significance of both health to identity and diet to health had so greatly expanded; and because of the dynamic interplay of prejudice against race, class, and body size, fatness undermined life chances in a way that bad eating habits never had. The fat-acceptance activist Marilyn Wann describes weight-based discrimination as "a cradle to grave phenomenon" and lists hundreds of studies documenting the impact of anti-fat attitudes. She points to research showing that fat children were sub-

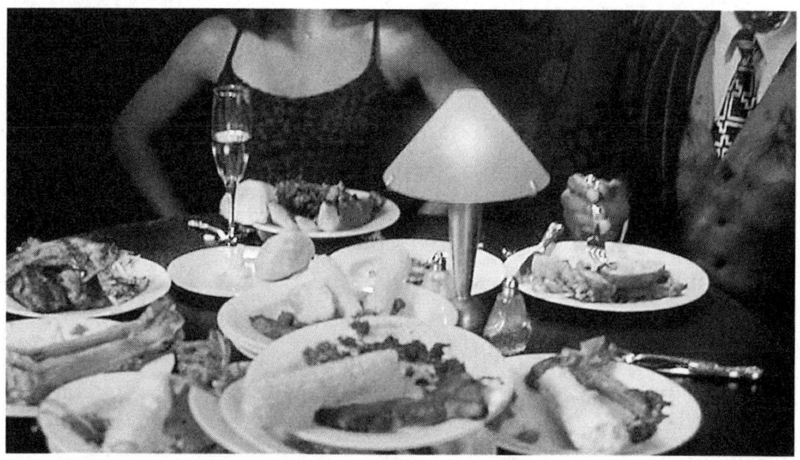

FIGURE 5.10 • Dinner at the comedy club. Still from *The Nutty Professor* (1996).

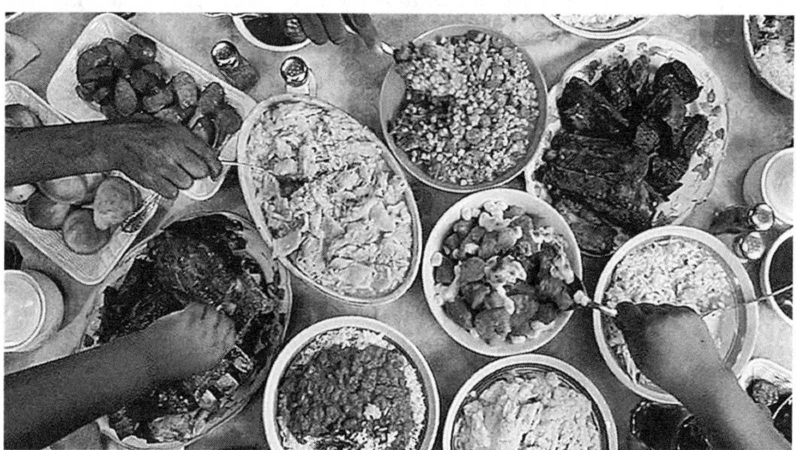

FIGURE 5.11 • Dinner at the Klump residence. Still from *The Nutty Professor* (1996).

jected to ridicule, ostracism, and discouragement from nursery school through college. Workplace discrimination was also found to be rampant: fat people were less likely to be hired (93 percent of human-resources professionals would prefer to hire a "normal weight" applicant) and earned less when they were (fat women earned $7,000 less per year than did thinner women). Studies showed fat people were less likely to be married and more likely to be socially isolated. Others showed that inadequate medical equipment, such as CT scans with weight limits, and biased attitudes among providers (who, for example, were less likely to conduct diagnostic exams that required touching a patient if the patient was fat) compromised their health.[134]

The stigma generated by obesity discourse also threatened the well-being of fat people by bringing into question whether or not they possessed the qualities of self that were seen as essential to moral personhood and good citizenship. At the core of this stigma lay the equivalence between thinness and self-control, which was considered a foundation of mature personhood and good citizenship. If fatness stood for a lack of self-control, then it also suggested that the fat person was not qualified for the rights and privileges of full personhood. Many fat people were painfully aware of this reality. One fat woman described starting school at age five and becoming for the first time "aware of the strange power of the word FAT" and the threat it posed to her very personhood. "There was," she recalls, "so clearly a consensus around me that being fat negated me as a valid human being."[135] It was in part the serious social threat posed by this negation that made weight loss such an important goal for "overweight" Americans in the early twenty-first century. As Wann argues, "People who say that they want to lose weight are speaking in code." What "seekers of weight loss truly desire," she explains, are "happiness, respect, full personhood, and minimization of physical and emotional suffering."[136]

ALTHOUGH IT WAS a public-health movement aimed at improving the health of the population, the campaign against obesity seriously threatened the well-being of the very people it purported to help. Its focus on the body as a moral measure produced a kind of stigma for those who (apparently) failed to live by the rules of dietary health that was far more vicious than anything that had previously accrued to the figure of the "bad eater." Although it was not about eating right in the strictest sense, the antiobesity campaign nonetheless exemplified the cultural politics of dietary reform in its extreme. Its empirical language of medical and scientific norms was a conduit for a powerful set of moral rules that were rarely questioned, even when they were noticed. Its messages conveyed an education in the cultural expectations of good citizenship and protected the ever-imperiled social boundaries of class and race in America. Most strikingly, as the most powerful discourse on food and health at the start of the twenty-first century, the antiobesity movement capitalized on and expanded the century of growth in the purview of dietary politics traced in this book. It demanded that every American take seriously the mandate to eat right, but extended the responsibility for dietary health across almost every facet of daily life, and did so within a political and social context in which practices of health were more central to the achievement of moral personhood and good citizenship than ever before.

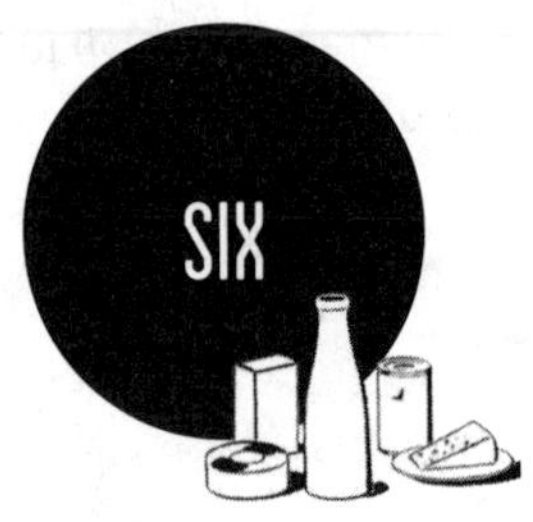

CONNECTING THE DOTS

Dietary Reform Past, Present, and Future

Not long before I finished writing this book, I found myself at a podium at the Whitten Building in Washington, the home of the U.S. Department of Agriculture (USDA). The room was full of university and USDA scientists involved in cutting-edge research on the relationship between diet and human health, hoping to give rise to a new nutritional paradigm. Collectively, the scientists, from the United States and Denmark, were amassing a set of tools that would replace dietary advice based on population averages with targeted interventions based on an individual's unique "phenotype," a composite of genetic, metabolic, microbial, and other measures. After two days of presentations on nutrigenomics, microbiomics, metabolomics, and sensory science, I had a chance to try to convince the people in that room to take seriously the cultural aspects of dietary health and to learn from the dietary reformers of the past. The challenge was to connect the dots between history and the present in a way that mattered for dietary reformers themselves.[1]

How *does* the history of dietary reform matter for dietary reformers, and the rest of us? What are the connections between the past, the present, and the future that matter for anyone who thinks about food and health? My arguments in this book don't add up to a revolutionary new way to eat right or to change people's eating habits, but they do suggest a new way of thinking about what dietary health is and means. Connecting the dots, in this case, may lead to more questions than answers, but changing the kinds of questions we ask is its own kind of revolution.

First, returning to that USDA conference room, I think through what the history I have written here can bring to dietary reform in the present. Then I think beyond dietary reformers, to consider how this history matters for all of us, starting with the big "us" of society. The history of the cultural politics of dietary health should cause us to ask some hard questions about the way we define and pursue health today. This history also presents an opportunity for a new kind of "dietary reform": not teaching people to eat right, but teaching the kind of critical thinking skills that, in light of the cultural politics of food and health revealed here, we all need. I end by considering the responsibility that a better understanding of the cultural content of dietary discourse implies for all of us, especially those of us who can and do "eat right."

For my talk at the USDA, I distilled lessons from the past into a series of provocations designed to help my colleagues understand the challenges they face as dietary reformers in the present. My intention was to introduce history as a tool critical to the success of dietary reform because it shows how deeply cultural the processes of defining a good diet and trying to change people's eating habits really are. My basic message was this: it's not enough to have fantastically innovative scientific insights and strategies. It's not even enough to take values, culture, and politics into consideration when figuring out how to best package and deliver new advice and strategies. Since, as history shows, the concept of dietary health is inseparable from cultural values, dietary reformers need to be reflexive about the cultural content of the ideals they promote, cautious about the moral implications of their discourse, and strategic about the values their lessons in eating right express. They must understand that dietary health has meaning and content that exists outside of what they have discovered in the lab, and that only by comprehending and working in concert with those meanings can they assure that the knowledge they produce has a beneficial impact. While such awareness certainly complicates their efforts, reformers are surely capable of grappling with these complexities. Furthermore, knowledge of history doesn't actually increase complexity—it sheds light on complexity that is already there. Nutrition reformers must inevitably deal with both the empirical and the ethical aspects of dietary health, and my hope is that this history helps illuminate the ethical implications of their work.

Learning from history can help dietary reformers meet their own goals. Most of the nutrition reformers that I know are especially concerned about the health implications of the diets of America's poor and underprivileged populations, and very frustrated about how hard it is to reach them. They want answers, but rarely look to history to provide them. History shows that class has historically been inseparable from the endeavor of dietary reform, that the dynamics of class and race both precede and motivate the impulse among middle- and upper-middle-class reformers to improve the eating habits of people of color and the poor. Today's reformers are unlikely to dismantle the nutritional class hierarchy without a concerted effort to find new approaches to reform. Furthermore, they are unlikely to improve eating habits among disadvantaged groups if their work continues to reproduce the dynamics of class at play throughout the last century. Understanding that dietary advice has historically contributed to the ongoing process of constructing the identity and status of the American middle and upper middle classes gives present-day reformers a chance, at least, to sidestep the pitfalls of the past. The history of dietary reform suggests that they should start by jettisoning the assumption that health has an essential, universal meaning, and that they should explore in earnest what health really means to the people whose diets they are trying to improve. As other critics have suggested, breaking free of history will require imagining and exploring new ways of promoting reform—not through better marketing, but through a process of determining aims and strategies that incorporates the perspectives of those who have historically been positioned as "unhealthy others."[2]

Dietary reformers can't teach people to "eat right" unless they understand and honor what "eating right" actually means, that is, not what a good diet comprises, but what it stands for. This is as true for those reformers who are driven by concerns about sustainability, social justice, and the food system as it is for those driven by nutrition science. Many concerned reformers have turned their attention to issues of access and equity in the food system. Working with a definition of a good diet that incorporates the fundamentals of nutrition and the ethics of alternative food, they are trying to combat diet-related health problems among the poor by making "good food" (fresh, local, organic produce) more accessible. Alternative food is driven by the fundamental conviction that eating is an agricultural, ethical, and political act, but *defining* a good diet is also inevitably a social, political, and moral act. Like science-driven reformers, social-justice-oriented reformers inherit a history of moralized class dynamics. They, too, should assume that they do not know what health really means to the people they are trying to reform, and they should consider not just pragmatic but also social and cultural factors that act as barriers to access to good food.[3] Are they, for example, working with a culturally biased definition of good food or dietary health that alienates the people they are trying to reach? In addition to economic and spatial barriers, does the historical relationship between the middle class, dietary reform, and eating right also act as a barrier to access to healthy food? My research into the discourses of dietary reform raises, but does not answer, these and many other questions about the experiences of the targets of dietary reform, both past and present. I hope that other researchers will fill out the limited picture I have painted and, especially, give voice to those people I have referred to as the "unhealthy other."

What about the bigger questions about "reform working"? While this history provides lessons that are useful for the project of dietary reform, it also raises important questions about that project. I hope this book sparks a conversation about the implications of our increasingly obsessive focus on diet as a source of biomedical health and social well-being. What does it reinforce, obscure, or occlude? Are we really talking about health when we talk about diet? As the purview and significance of dietary health expands, we are redefining health in the image of diet. The importance of diet as a health determinant emerged from the postwar shift to lifestyle as the primary means through which practices of health were organized. The late-twentieth-century expansion of the social significance of eating right reflects the growing emphasis on individual behavior. But the role of dietary discourse may also be to further inflate our sense of the individual's capacity to control his or her biology and to take responsibility for that body's productive potential or, conversely, its potential as a drag on public resources. The more we talk about putting the lid on the cookie jar as a means of securing the nation's social stability or economic viability, the less we talk about the other issues that comprise both individual health and social and economic well-being.[4] I believe that people have a right to adequate, nourishing, and pleasurable food, and I do not discount the biomedical and social value of the pursuit of dietary health for those who promote it or attempt to attain it by eating right. But I also believe that we as a society owe it to ourselves to engage in a critical reappraisal of the results of our obsession with diet as a proxy for health. I am not sure that we are talking about the health that we really want when we talk about eating habits; diet talk too often obscures structural and environmental stresses, constraints, exposures, and inequities, while naturalizing the dubious redefinition of health as an individual responsibility and imperative.

In addition to the big questions about the social role of dietary discourse, *Eating Right* also suggests some questions we can all ask in the face of the dietary advice that we encounter day to day. When we see or hear dietary advice, we should consider both its empirical and its ethical aspects. History shows that rules about what to eat are at the same time guidelines for becoming a moral person and a good citizen. Given this, being an informed consumer of dietary advice requires more than a working knowledge of nutrition. Others have pointed out that skepticism about the ideology of nutrition, or nutritionism, is also required, that people should learn to assess and value qualities of food beyond what nutrition can measure.[5] Critics have also argued that consumers of dietary advice should be very careful about confusing marketing with sound nutritional advice, and that people should be cognizant of the food industry's role in shaping even the USDA's nutrition guidelines.[6] I agree, but I would add that being an informed consumer also requires thinking critically about dietary advice as a cultural construction.

Knowing what we now know about the cultural politics of dietary health, we should all ask ourselves certain questions when confronted with dietary advice that have nothing to do with scientific veracity or industry influence, ones that emphasize the social role of dietary advice over its actual content. This brings me back to the shock I experienced at discovering that while Alice Waters promoted ideas about a good diet that were radically different from those espoused by Ellen Richards, the two reformers were motivated by unexpectedly similar beliefs about the social role and significance of eating right. Fundamental assumptions about the social role of eating right are embedded in every dietary recommendation, and our job as consumers is to become aware of those assumptions so that we can engage with them intentionally, rather than haphazardly. Understanding that talking about dietary health is inevitably talking about social values, morality, ideals of good citizenship, and class can motivate us to pay more attention to all of our entanglements with ideas about eating right. Perhaps we need to establish and promote a new set of competencies for interpreting the ethical aspects of dietary advice. Like media literacy, "dietary literacy" would start with the assumption that all messages are constructed and have a purpose beyond the communication of nutritional facts. It would teach people to think about the ethical conveyed in the empirical, to decipher the social norms, moral implications, and class dynamics embedded in all messages about what is good to eat.[7]

With awareness comes accountability. Jay Mechling, my former colleague in the American Studies Program at the University of California, Davis, has written eloquently about the role that cultural criticism can play, explaining that its goal should be to make people's lives better by giving them the opportunity to arrive at their "everyday practices by choice, not by uncritical inheritance."[8] For those of us who can and do choose to "eat right," understanding the cultural politics of dietary health presents a particular kind of call to awareness and accountability. Given its social and moral freight, eating right is a kind of unexamined social privilege. It is not unlike and is clearly connected to other forms of privilege that usually go unnoticed by the people who possess them, such as whiteness and thinness. Choosing socially sanctioned diets makes subtle but very powerful claims to morality, responsibility, and fitness for good citizenship. We who are lucky enough to have eating habits that align with dietary ideals or inhabit the kind of bodies that imply we do may think that our shapes or healthy preferences are a sign of our virtue, the result of our will, or perhaps nothing more than a lucky twist of fate, but history shows that there are cultural mechanisms that produce the seemingly natural alignment between ideal diets, ideal body sizes, and the habits and preferences of the elite. We should therefore question our common-sense assumptions about the "goodness" of good eaters and be very careful about the subtle forms of social and moral condemnation we mete out, often unconsciously, to "bad eaters." I am not suggesting that those of us who "eat right" should turn away from habits we find pleasurable, healthy, and just, but I do hope that we might begin to notice the social role our eating habits and our ideas about good food inevitably play.

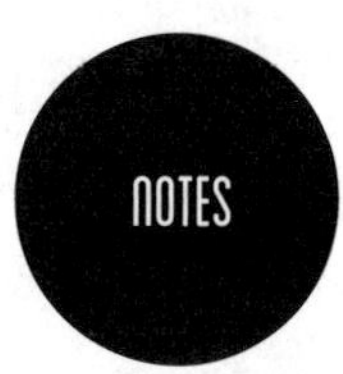

ONE
The Cultural Politics of Dietary Health

The epigraphs are drawn from, respectively, Ellen Richards, *Euthenics: The Science of a Controllable Environment* (Boston: Whitcomb and Barrows, 1910), 100; Consumer Counsel Division of the U.S. Department of Agriculture, "Food and National Defense Issue," *Consumer's Guide* 6, no. 20 (1943); Molly O'Neill, "Keeper of the Flame," *New York Times Magazine*, December 12, 1992, 29; Richard Carmona, "Remarks at the American Enterprise Institute Obesity Conference," U.S. Department of Health and Human Services, Washington, D.C., June 10, 2003.

1. Laura Shapiro, *Perfection Salad: Women and Cooking at the Turn of the Century* (New York: Henry Holt and Company, 1986).

2. This argument draws on the theory of class developed by Pierre Bourdieu, in *Distinction: A Social Critique of the Judgment of Taste* (Cambridge, MA: Harvard University Press, 1984).

3. Joan Burbick, *Healing the Republic: The Language of Health and the Culture of Nationalism in Nineteenth-Century America* (Cambridge: Cambridge University Press, 1994), 17.

4. Robert Crawford, "A Cultural Account of 'Health': Control, Release, and the Social Body," in *Issues on the Political Economy of Health Care*, ed. John B. McKinley (New York: Tavistock Publications, 1984), 62.

5. Crawford, "A Cultural Account of 'Health.'"

6. John Coveney, *Food, Morals, and Meaning: The Pleasure and Anxiety of Eating* (New York: Routledge, 2000), 63.

7. See Charlotte Biltekoff, "Critical Nutrition Studies," in *Handbook of Food History*, ed. Jeffrey Pilcher (New York: Oxford, 2012), for a more developed exploration of the historiography of nutrition and the emergence of "critical nutrition studies." See the following for more on the two "key insights" of critical nutrition studies: Deborah Lupton, *Food, the Body and the Self* (London: Sage, 1996); Deborah Lupton

and Alan Petersen, *The New Public Health: Health and Self in the Age of Risk* (London: Sage, 1996); Coveney, *Food, Morals, and Meaning*; Nick Cullather, "The Foreign Policy of the Calorie," *American Historical Review* 112, no. 2 (2007); Jessica Mudry, *Measured Meals: Nutrition in America* (Albany: SUNY Press, 2009); Gyorgy Scrinis, "On the Ideology of Nutritionism," *Gastronomic* 8, no. 1 (2008); Gyorgy Scrinis, *Nutritionism: The Science and Politics of Dietary Advice* (New York: Columbia University Press, 2013).

8. For an excellent overview of the field, see Sondra Solovay and Esther Rothblum, eds., *The Fat Studies Reader* (New York: NYU Press, 2009); Jana Evans Braziel and Kathleen LeBesco, eds., *Bodies Out of Bounds: Fatness and Transgression* (Berkeley: University of California Press, 2001).

9. For more on this history, see Coveney, *Food, Morals, and Meaning*. See also Stephen Nissenbaum, *Sex, Diet, and Debility in Jacksonian America: Sylvester Graham and Health Reform* (Westport, CT: Greenwood Press, 1980); James C. Whorton, *Crusaders for Fitness: The History of American Health Reformers* (Princeton, NJ: Princeton University Press, 1982).

10. Charles E. Rosenberg, *No Other Gods: On Science and American Social Thought* (Baltimore: Johns Hopkins University Press, 1961); Harmke Kamminga and Andrew Cunningham, "Introduction: The Science and Culture of Nutrition, 1840–1940," in *The Science and Culture of Nutrition, 1840–1940*, ed. Harmke Kamminga and Andrew Cunningham (Amsterdam: Rodopi, 1995), 13.

11. Robert Crawford, "The Boundaries of the Self and the Unhealthy Other: Reflections on Health, Culture and AIDS," *Social Science Medicine* 38, no. 10 (1994).

12. Patricia Allen, *Together at the Table: Sustainability and Sustenance in the American Agrifood System* (University Park: Pennsylvania State University Press/Rural Sociological Society, 2004), 6.

TWO
Scientific Moralization and the Beginning of Modern Dietary Reform

1. See U.S. Department of Agriculture, ChooseMyPlate.gov, available at http://www.choosemyplate.gov/.

2. The politics behind nutritional recommendations are covered in Marion Nestle, *Food Politics: How the Food Industry Influences Nutrition and Health* (Berkeley: University of California Press, 2002).

3. Harvey Levenstein, *Revolution at the Table: The Transformation of the American Diet* (New York: Oxford University Press, 1988); Laura Shapiro, *Perfection Salad: Women and Cooking at the Turn of the Century* (New York: Henry Holt, 1986); Warren Belasco, "Food, Morality, and Social Reform," in *Morality and Health*, ed. Paul Rozin and Allen M. Brandt (New York: Routledge, 1997).

4. John Coveney, *Food, Morals, and Meaning: The Pleasure and Anxiety of Eating* (New York: Routledge, 2000), 53–56.

5. For more on the politics and ideology of nutritional quantification, particularly at the USDA, see Jessica Mudry, *Measured Meals: Nutrition in America* (Albany: SUNY Press, 2009).

6. Levenstein, *Revolution at the Table*, 46.

7. Charles E. Rosenberg, *No Other Gods: On Science and American Social Thought* (Baltimore: Johns Hopkins University Press, 1961), 20.

8. W. O. Atwater and Charles Woods, *The Chemical Composition of American Food Materials* (Washington, DC: U.S. Department of Agriculture, Office of Experiment Stations, 1899).

9. Harvey Levenstein, *Paradox of Plenty: A Social History of Eating in Modern America* (New York: Oxford University Press, 1993), 97.

10. Levenstein, *Revolution at the Table*; Mudry, *Measured Meals*.

11. Coveney argues that Atwater's work defined poor choices about what to eat not only as physiologically foolish but also as morally problematic and that his work was therefore a good example of "modern nutrition functioning as an empirical science *and* a spiritual discipline." Coveney, *Food, Morals, and Meaning*, 62. In *Measured Meals* Jessica Mudry describes Atwater's work as conflating quality and quantity, therefore providing a way by which the "quality of an eater could be judged easily or compared on the basis of caloric or nutritive content of their diet." As she points out, Atwater's quantification of American food objectified "once-moralistic terms like 'good' and 'bad,'" while giving the USDA the terms and technologies to promote "gastro-fiscal responsibility" and "dietary morality." Mudry, *Measured Meals*, 42, 43.

12. Wilbur O. Atwater, "Pecuniary Economy of Food: The Chemistry of Foods and Nutrition V," *Century*, November 1887–April 1888, 445.

13. Atwater, "Pecuniary Economy of Food," 445.

14. Atwater, "Pecuniary Economy of Food," 445.

15. Atwater, "Pecuniary Economy of Food," 445.

16. Atwater, "Pecuniary Economy of Food," 437.

17. Atwater, "Pecuniary Economy of Food," 445.

18. Rosenberg, *No Other Gods*, 3, 10.

19. Mudry, *Measured Meals*, 10; Daniel Patrick Thurs, *Science Talk: Changing Notions of Science in American Culture* (New Brunswick, NJ: Rutgers University Press, 2008), 4, 11. Charles Rosenberg explains, "Every culture needs to create and communicate an appropriate social ideology and in doing so must draw upon those sources of authority clothed with the greatest emotional relevance," such as science (Rosenberg, *No Other Gods*, 2).

20. Rosenberg, *No Other Gods*, 12. In his book about the social-hygiene movements of the late nineteenth century, David Pivar writes, "Hygienic and dietary reforms acquired eschatological meaning and became pregnant with moral purpose." David Pivar, *Purity Crusade: Sexual Morality and Social Control, 1868–1900* (Westport, CT: Greenwood Press, 1973), 171.

21. Barbara Leslie Epstein, *The Politics of Domesticity: Women, Evangelism, and Temperance in Nineteenth-Century America* (Middletown, CT: Wesleyan University Press, 1981); Lori D. Ginzberg, *Women and the Work of Benevolence: Morality, Politics and Class in the Nineteenth-Century United States* (New Haven, CT: Yale University Press, 1990); Pivar, *Purity Crusade*.

22. Irma Jones, "Ethics of the Kitchen," *New England Kitchen*, December 1894, 109, 112.

23. Jones, "Ethics of the Kitchen," 122.

24. Mary L. Wade, "Healthful and Economical Foods," *New England Kitchen*, April 1896, 33.

25. Helen Ekin Starrett, "The Home and the Labor Problem," *New England Kitchen*, February 1895, 241.

26. Maude H. Lacy, "A Neglected Side of the Labor Problem." *American Kitchen Magazine*, November 1899, 45.

27. Isabel Bevier, "Mrs. Richards' Relation to the Home Economics Movement," *Journal of Home Economics*, June 1911, 214.

28. Ellen Richards, *The Art of Right Living* (Boston: Whitcomb and Barrows, 1904), 16.

29. Shapiro, *Perfection Salad*, 129.

30. Cities in which studies were conducted include Chicago, New York, and Pittsburg. Colleges at which studies were conducted include Purdue University, Main State College, and the University of Tennessee.

31. Isabel Bevier, "The U.S. Government and the Housewife," *American Kitchen*, December 1898.

32. Bevier, "The U.S. Government and the Housewife."

33. W. O. Atwater and Charles D. Woods, *Dietary Studies in New York City in 1895 and 1896, Bulletin No. 46*, edited by U.S. Department of Agriculture Office of Experiment Stations (Washington, DC: U.S. Government Printing Office, 1898), 10.

34. For an exploration of how the calorie made it possible to compare diets of different nations and the implications for American foreign policy, see Nick Cullather, "The Foreign Policy of the Calorie." *American Historical Review* 112, no. 2 (2007), 337–64.

35. W. T. Sedgwick, "On External Digestion Commonly Called Alimentation," *The Rumford Kitchen Leaflets: Plain Words About Food*, ed. Ellen Richards (Boston: Home Science Publishing, 1899), 45.

36. Sedgwick, "On External Digestion Commonly Called Alimentation," 49.

37. Coveney, *Food, Morals, and Meaning*, 63.

38. R. H. Chittenden, "The Digestibility of Proteid Foods," in *The Rumford Kitchen Leaflets: Plain Words about Food*, ed. Ellen H. Richards (Boston: Home Science Publishing, 1899).

39. Ellen Richards, "Good Food For Little Money," *The Rumford Kitchen Leaflets: Plain Words about Food*, ed. Ellen Richards (Boston: Home Science Publishing, 1899), 124; Ellen Richards, *The Cost of Food: A Study of Dietaries* (New York: J. Wiley and Sons, 1901), 20.

40. Richards, *The Cost of Food*, 20.

41. Mary Hinman Abel, "King Palate," *The Rumford Kitchen Leaflets: Plain Words About Food*, ed. Ellen Richards (Boston: Home Science Publishing, 1899).

42. More branches were later opened in Boston, one in the primarily black West End and another in the ethnically diverse North End. Eventually, kitchens were also established in Chicago and New York, as well as in conjunction with the Philadelphia College Settlement House. See Levenstein, *Revolution at the Table*, 50–52.

43. Caroline L. Hunt, *The Life of Ellen Richards* (Boston: Whitcomb and Barrows, 1912), 218.

44. Mary Hinman Abel, "The Story of the New England Kitchen: Part 2, A Study in Social Economics," *The Rumford Kitchen Leaflets: Plain Words about Food*, ed. Ellen Richards (Boston: Home Science Publishing, 1899), 149; Hunt, *The Life of Ellen Richards*, 219.

45. Abel, "The Story of the New England Kitchen," 137.

46. Maria Parloa, "The New England Kitchen," *Century*, December 1891, 317.

47. Levenstein, *Revolution at the Table*, 54.

48. Hunt, *The Life of Ellen Richards*, 220.

49. For a discussion of why and how taste, tradition, and culture might be reincorporated into prevailing notions of good food, see Mudry, *Measured Meals*, chap. 5.

50. Levenstein, *Revolution at the Table*, 56.

51. For an elaboration and explication of this argument, see Coveney, *Food, Morals, and Meaning*.

52. Sarah Stage, "Ellen Richards and the Social Significance of the Home Economics Movement," *Rethinking Home Economics: Women and the History of a Profession*, ed. Sarah Stage and Virginia B. Vincenti (Ithaca, NY: Cornell University Press, 1997), 25–26.

53. Lake Placid Conference on Home Economics, *Proceedings of the First, Second, and Third Conferences* (Lake Placid, NY: American Home Economics Association, 1899–1901).

54. Henrietta Goodrich, "Suggestions for a Professional School of Home and Social Economics," in *Proceedings of the First, Second, and Third Conferences*, by Lake Placid Conference on Home Economics (Lake Placid, NY: American Home Economics Association, 1899–1901).

55. Shapiro, *Perfection Salad*, 185–86.

56. As the historian Sarah Stage argues, Richards's home economics emphasized municipal housekeeping and formed an important part of women's political culture in the Progressive Era. According to Stage the movement was not, as others have suggested, about keeping women in the home; it expanded women's political power and created a way for women to participate in the social activism of Progressive reform. Stage, "Ellen Richards and the Social Significance of the Home Economics Movement," 18, 28.

57. Hunt, *The Life of Ellen Richards*, 233–34.

58. James C. Whorton, *Crusaders for Fitness: The History of American Health Reformers* (Princeton, NJ: Princeton University Press, 1982), 163; Howard Horowitz, "Always with Us," *American Literary History* 10, no. 2 (summer 1998).

59. Whorton, *Crusaders for Fitness*, 163–64.

60. Kathy J. Cooke, "The Limits of Heredity: Nature and Nurture in American Eugenics before 1915," *Journal of the History of Biology* 31 (1998), 266.

61. Richards, *The Cost of Food*, 9.

62. Ellen Richards, "Nomenclature," in *Proceedings of the Sixth Conference*, by Lake Placid Conference on Home Economics (Lake Placid, NY: American Home Economics Association, 1904), 63.

63. Ellen Richards, "Euthenics in Higher Education: Better Living Conditions," in

Proceedings of the Eighth Conference, by Lake Placid Conference on Home Economics (Lake Placid, NY: American Home Economics Association, 1906), 33.

64. Ellen Richards, *Euthenics: The Science of a Controllable Environment* (Boston: Whitcomb and Barrows, 1910), vii.

65. Richards, *Euthenics*, vii.

66. Richards, *Euthenics*, viii.

67. Richards, *Euthenics*, 100.

68. Stage, "Ellen Richards and the Social Significance of the Home Economics Movement," 27.

69. Lake Placid Conference on Home Economics, *Proceedings of the Sixth Conference* (Lake Placid, NY: American Home Economics Association, 1904), 64.

70. Richards, *The Art of Right Living*, 65, 47–48.

71. This is not to be confused with the system of law, also called natural law, that is used to deduce rules of moral behavior.

72. Lake Placid Conference on Home Economics, *Proceedings of the First, Second, and Third Conferences*, 14.

73. Hazel T. Craig, *The History of Home Economics* (New York: Practical Home Economics, 1946).

74. Ellen Richards, "Social Significance of the Home Economics Movement," *Journal of Home Economics* 3, no. 2 (1911), 122.

75. Robert H. Weibe, *The Search for Order, 1877–1920* (New York: Hill and Wang, 1967), 159; Joan Burbick, *Healing the Republic: The Language of Health and the Culture of Nationalism in Nineteenth-Century America* (Cambridge: Cambridge University Press, 1994), 302.

76. Weibe, *The Search for Order*, 159.

77. Burbick, *Healing the Republic*, 302.

78. Mary Hinman Abel, "Proteid or Albuminous Food in Our Daily Fare," *The Rumford Kitchen Leaflets: Plain Words about Food*, ed. Ellen Richards (Boston: Home Science Publishing, 1899), 68.

79. Abel, "Proteid or Albuminous Food in Our Daily Fare," 31, 161.

80. Julie A. Reuben, "Beyond Politics: Community Civics and the Redefinition of Citizenship in the Progressive Era," *History of Education Quarterly* 37, no. 4 (winter 1997), 418–19.

81. Reuben, "Beyond Politics," 416.

82. Richards, *Euthenics*, 134–35.

83. Lake Placid Conference on Home Economics, *Proceedings of the First, Second, and Third Conferences*, 30.

84. Richards, *Euthenics*, 40.

85. Richards, *Euthenics*, 41.

86. Richards, *The Cost of Food*, 7.

87. Richards, *The Cost of Food*, 7.

88. Richards, *The Cost of Food*, 7.

89. Richards, *The Cost of Food*, 6.

90. Lake Placid Conference on Home Economics, *Proceedings of the Fourth Conference* (Lake Placid, NY: American Home Economics Association, 1902), 35.

91. Lake Placid Conference on Home Economics, *Proceedings of the First, Second, and Third Conferences*, 4.

92. Lake Placid Conference on Home Economics, *Proceedings of the First, Second, and Third Conferences*, 4.

93. "Foods Prepared and Sold at the Rumford Kitchen, with Their Food Values," in *The Rumford Kitchen Leaflets: Plain Words about Food*, ed. Ellen Richards (Boston: Home Science Publishing, 1899).

94. "Guide to the Rumford Kitchen," in *The Rumford Kitchen Leaflets: Plain Words about Food*, ed. Ellen Richards (Boston: Home Science Publishing, 1899), 12, 14.

95. Ellen Richards, ed., *The Rumford Kitchen Leaflets: Plain Words about Food* (Boston: Home Science Publishing, 1899).

96. Stuart M. Blumin, *The Emergence of the Middle Class: Social Experience in the American City, 1760–1900* (Cambridge: Cambridge University Press, 1989), 297.

97. Weibe, *The Search for Order*, 13.

98. Blumin, *The Emergence of the Middle Class*, 290–96; Samuel P. Hays, *The Response to Industrialism 1885–1914*, 2d ed. (Chicago: University of Chicago Press, 1995), 99.

99. Robert Crawford, "The Boundaries of the Self and the Unhealthy Other: Reflections on Health, Culture and AIDS," *Social Science Medicine* 38, no. 10 (1994), 1348.

100. Nancy Tomes, "Moralizing the Microbe: The Germ Theory and the Moral Construction of Behavior in the Late-Nineteenth-Century Antituberculosis Movement," in *Morality and Health*, ed. Allen M. Brandt and Paul Rozin (New York: Routledge, 1997), 288.

101. The leaflets also included, among other things, lessons on the chemistry of food and digestion, advice about feeding schoolchildren and the ill, and the allegorical tale of "King Palate." Richards, *The Rumford Kitchen Leaflets*.

102. Mary Hinman Abel, "Public Kitchens in Relation to Workingmen and the Average Housewife," in *The Rumford Kitchen Leaflets: Plain Words about Food*, ed. Ellen Richards (Boston: Home Science Publishing, 1899), 159.

103. This refers to Pierre Bourdieu's concept of "habitus," or necessity internalized and converted into a disposition that generates meaningful practices and meaning-giving perceptions. Pierre Bourdieu, *Distinction: A Social Critique of the Judgment of Taste* (Cambridge, MA: Harvard University Press, 1984).

104. Richards, *The Cost of Food*, 2.

105. Abel, "Proteid or Albuminous Food in Our Daily Fare," 68.

106. Richards, *The Cost of Food*, 138, 11.

107. Ethel Davis, "Dishonesty in Caste and in House-furnishing," *New England Kitchen*, September 1894, 269.

108. Ethel Davis, "Dishonesty and Caste in Housekeeping and Home-making," *New England Kitchen*, January 1895, 172.

109. W. O. Atwater, "How Food Nourishes the Body: The Chemistry of Food and Nutrition II," *Century*, May–October 1887, 251.

110. Atwater, "How Food Nourishes the Body," 251.

111. Anna Barrows, "The Provision of Food for a Typical American Family," *American Kitchen*, October 1896, 28.

112. Ellen Richards, "The Foods of Institutions," in *The Rumford Kitchen Leaflets: Plain Words about Food*, ed. Ellen Richards (Boston: Home Science Publishing, 1899), 168.

113. Richards, *The Cost of Food*, 37–44.

114. Jonathan Kasson argues that the elaborate table manners detailed by etiquette writers at the time played an important social role, imposing rank and establishing order in an increasingly fluid and pluralistic society. Eventually, however, such manners became naturalized, seeming to set the classes apart on the basis of "natural" differences in behavior and bodily comportment which were, in reality, purely cultural. John F. Kasson, "Rituals of Dining: Table Manners in Victorian America," in *Dining in America, 1850–1900*, ed. Kathryn Grover (Rochester, NY: Margaret Woodbury Strong Museum, 1987).

115. Kasson, "Rituals of Dining," 77–83.

116. Kasson, "Rituals of Dining," 77–83.

117. Bourdieu, *Distinction*.

118. Thurs, *Science Talk*, 4, 11; Mudry, *Measured Meals*, 6.

119. Gyorgy Scrinis, "On the Ideology of Nutritionism," *Gastronomic* 8, no. 1 (2008).

120. Michael Pollan, *In Defense of Food: An Eater's Manifesto* (New York: Penguin, 2008).

THREE

Anxiety and Aspiration on the Nutrition Front

1. The nine hundred invited delegates included experts on dietary reform (professional nutritionists, home economists, educators, physicians, public health officers, and social workers) and representatives of a variety of vested sectors: industry, labor and the government; the press and the radio; colleges, universities and medical schools; farm organizations; consumer groups; and processing and marketing organizations. *Proceedings of the National Nutrition Conference for Defense* (Washington, DC: Federal Security Agency, Office of the Director of Defense, Health and Welfare Services, 1941).

2. *Proceedings of the National Nutrition Conference for Defense*, 1.

3. Helen Veit argues that the food campaign responded to concerns that Americans had grown physically and spiritually lax since the Civil War by promoting the renunciation of food pleasure as a patriotic duty. Helen Zoe Veit, "'We Were a Soft People': Asceticism, Self-Discipline and American Food Conservation in the First World War," *Food, Culture and Society* 10, no. 2 (summer 2007), 180.

4. Harvey Levenstein, *Revolution at the Table: The Transformation of the American Diet* (New York: Oxford University Press, 1988), 146.

5. Levenstein, *Revolution at the Table*, 148.

6. Levenstein, *Revolution at the Table*, 148, 152–53.

7. "Superflour," *New York Times*, January 12, 1941.

8. Harvey Levenstein, *Paradox of Plenty: A Social History of Eating in Modern America* (New York: Oxford University Press, 1993), 57–58.

9. Food and Nutrition Board Committee on Diagnosis and Pathology of Nutritional Deficiencies, "Inadequate Diets and Nutritional Deficiencies in the United States: Their Prevalence and Significance," in *Bulletin of the National Research Council No. 109* (Washington, DC: National Research Council, National Academy of Sciences, 1943).

10. Hazel Stiebeling, "Family Food Consumption and Dietary Levels: Five Regions," in *U.S. Department of Agriculture Misc. Pub. no. 405* (Washington, DC: U.S. Government Printing Office, 1941).

11. Levenstein, *Paradox of Plenty*, 54.

12. The earliest use of the term I have found is in an article translating a League of Nations nutrition report into practical recommendations for the homemaker: Florence Brobeck, "Protective Foods for the Family," *New York Times*, March 8, 1936.

13. Louise Stanley, "Science of Nutrition at the Home Base," in *The Family in a World at War*, ed. Sidonie Matsnder Gruenberg (New York: Harper Brothers, 1942), 46; available at http://hdl.handle.net/2027/coo.31924003554 96.

14. Levenstein, *Paradox of Plenty*, 59–60, 67–68.

15. *Proceedings of the National Nutrition Conference for Defense*, 4.

16. Alarm over hungry children and outrage over "breadlines knee deep in wheat" spurred periodic government concern about national nutrition during the Depression, but the economic and political constraints of the era prevented a dietary-reform movement from emerging. In 1933, for example, Secretary of Labor Frances Perkins received distressing reports from the Children's Bureau about rates of child malnutrition and called a special national conference in response to the crisis. Despite dramatic rhetoric about starving children at the conference, little was accomplished in terms of gaining federal support to help feed the hungry. Levenstein argues that the failure of the conference on child nutrition was typical of national efforts to deal with hunger during the decade. While distribution of food stocks accumulating under federal programs designed to maintain prices by purchasing supplies seemed the obvious solution, powerful farm interests and government administrators hampered every effort to do so. Nutrition education that may have helped people to make better use of limited supplies was also blocked by farmers concerned that the messages of dietary reformers might reduce consumption of some commodities. As Levenstein writes, "Paranoid farm interests pounced on [the] most timid steps in the direction of promoting dietary change." Levenstein, *Paradox of Plenty*, 53–56, 54.

17. Richard Osborn Cummings, *The American and His Food: A History of Food Habits in the United States* (Chicago: University of Chicago Press, 1940), 231.

18. *Proceedings of the National Nutrition Conference for Defense*, 64.

19. *Proceedings of the National Nutrition Conference for Defense*, 64.

20. *Proceedings of the National Nutrition Conference for Defense*, 64.

21. "McNutt Takes Up New Defense Task," *New York Times*, December 4, 1940.

22. Lydia J. Roberts, "Beginning of the Recommended Dietary Allowances," *Journal of the American Dietetic Association* 34, no. 9 (1958), 33.

23. The committee began by creating a tentative list of values for various nutrients based on a survey of all related research reports. This list was then approved through a year-long process of consensus and revision. After the committee had approved it, it was reviewed by nutrition workers throughout the country, revised according to their suggestions, reviewed by the FNB, and finally presented to the American Institute of Nutrition, where the recommendations were accepted; Roberts, "Beginning of the Recommended Dietary Allowances," 33.

The recommendations turned out to be very similar—except for increases in calcium, riboflavin, and thiamine—to those that had been used throughout the 1930s to assess the adequacy of diets. Cummings, *The American and His Food*, 233–34.

24. *Proceedings of the National Nutrition Conference for Defense*, ix.

25. Jessica Mudry points out that the RDAs were distinct from past USDA guides in that they not only enumerated food but also quantified the body's relationship to food. They "represent the moment in which the person, in the process of eating, falls away, and the judgment of the goodness of a meal and the goodness of an American becomes a measurement." Jessica Mudry, *Measured Meals: Nutrition in America* (Albany: SUNY Press, 2009), 64.

26. Levenstein, *Paradox of Plenty*, 66.

27. *Proceedings of the National Nutrition Conference for Defense*, 32.

28. *Proceedings of the National Nutrition Conference for Defense*, 37.

29. Levenstein, *Paradox of Plenty*, 150.

30. Food and Nutrition Board Committee on Diagnosis and Pathology of Nutritional Deficiencies, "Inadequate Diets and Nutritional Deficiencies in the United States," 13.

31. Food and Nutrition Board Committee on Diagnosis and Pathology of Nutritional Deficiencies, "Inadequate Diets and Nutritional Deficiencies in the United States," 1–3.

32. Food and Nutrition Board Committee on Diagnosis and Pathology of Nutritional Deficiencies, "Inadequate Diets and Nutritional Deficiencies in the United States," 1–3.

33. Food and Nutrition Board Committee on Diagnosis and Pathology of Nutritional Deficiencies, "Inadequate Diets and Nutritional Deficiencies in the United States," 20.

34. Food and Nutrition Board Committee on Diagnosis and Pathology of Nutritional Deficiencies, "Inadequate Diets and Nutritional Deficiencies in the United States," 20.

35. *Proceedings of the National Nutrition Conference for Defense*, 220.

36. *Proceedings of the National Nutrition Conference for Defense*, 2.

37. *Proceedings of the National Nutrition Conference for Defense*, 30.

38. *Proceedings of the National Nutrition Conference for Defense*, 219.

39. Karen Anderson, *Wartime Women: Sex Roles, Family Relations, and the Status of Women during World War II* (Westport, CT: Greenwood Press, 1981); Amy Bentley, *Eating for Victory: Food Rationing and the Politics of Domesticity* (Urbana: University of Illinois Press, 1998); Lawrence R. Samuel, *Pledging Allegiance: American Identity and the Bond Drive of World War II* (Washington, DC: Smithsonian Institution Press, 1997); Allan M. Winkler, *Home Front U.S.A.: America during World War Two* (Arlington Heights, IL: Harlan Davidson, 1986).

40. Amy Bentley argues that home-front food programs "helped instill in Americans a sense of public commitment to the war, community involvement, and patriotism." Messages about food helped to offset home-front rhetoric that focused on private material and familial interests, providing a more "communally oriented vision of America" that was important for wartime social cohesion and morale. Bentley, *Eating for Victory*, 3–4.

41. War Information Program, *Food Fights for Freedom*, report prepared by Office of Program Coordination, Office of War Information, and War Food Administration, in cooperation with Office of Price Administration, 1943.

42. War Information Program, *Food Fights for Freedom*, 39.

43. War Information Program, *Food Fights for Freedom*, 1–3.

44. Philip Gleason, "Pluralism, Democracy and Catholicism in the Era of World War II," *Review of Politcs* 49, no. 2 (1987), 220.

45. *Proceedings of the National Nutrition Conference for Defense*, 56–61.

46. U.S. Department of Agriculture, *Democracy Means All of Us* (Washington, DC: Federal Security Agency, Office of Defense Health and Welfare Services, 1943).

47. Many of these committees had been active since the fall and winter of 1940–41, when land-grant colleges were asked to establish state nutrition committees and set up machinery for the development of local programs. New York State College of Home Economics, Department of Food and Nutrition, "Newsletter no. 2, March 15 1941." "Records #23/14/2485," Division of Rare and Manuscript Collections, Cornell University. U.S. Department of Agriculture, *Democracy Means All of Us*.

48. "Newsletter no. 2, March 15 1941."

49. "Newsletter no. 2, March 15 1941."

50. "Newsletter no. 2, March 15 1941."

51. Marion Jordan Ulmer, "Feeding Four on a Dollar a Day" (Denver: Marion Jordon Ulmer, 1942).

52. *Report on Nutrition Activities 1941–1942* (Ithaca: New York State College of Home Economics, 1942), 3.

53. "Your Child's Eating Habits," New York State College of Agriculture Farm Radio Brief, Cornell University radio brief, June 19, 1941.

54. "Food First," Cornell University radio brief, August 21, 1941.

55. *Vitality Vigor Vim Vitamins for Victory: Plan for Vitamins Every Day*, New York State Nutrition Committee. (Cornell: NY State College of Home Economics), Collection #23–2–749 BOX #19.

56. General Mills, *General Mills Nutrition Study Kit* (Minneapolis: General Mills, 1941).

57. *Report on Nutrition Activities 1941–1942*, 3; "What Foods to Eat and Why" leader's outline, New York State College of Home Economics, Cornell University, October 3, 1941, filed with the *Report on Nutrition Activities 1941–1942*.

58. Carl E. Guthrie, "History of the Committee on Food Habits," in Committee on Food Habits, *The Problem of Changing Food Habits: Report of the Committee on Food Habits 1941–1943, Bulletin of the National Research Council No. 108* (Washington, DC: National Research Council, National Academy of Sciences, 1943), 9–19.

59. Committee on Food Habits, "Manual for the Study of Food Habits," in Report of the Committee on Food Habits (Washington, DC: National Research Council, 1945), 24–25. See also Committee on Food Habits, "The Problem of Changing Food Habits."

60. Mary Sweeny, "Changing Food Habits," *Journal of Home Economics* 43, no. 7 (1942), 459.

61. Committee on Food Habits, "Manual for the Study of Food Habits," 24–25; Margaret Mead, "The Problem of Changing Food Habits," in Committee on Food Habits, *The Problem of Changing Food Habits*, 20–31.

62. Committee on Food Habits, "Manual for the Study of Food Habits," 24–25.

63. William Graebner, *The Engineering of Consent: Democracy and Authority in Twentieth-Century America* (Madison: University of Wisconsin Press, 1987), 4–5.

64. Graebner, *The Engineering of Consent*, 104.

65. Kurt Lewin, "Forces behind Food Habits and Methods of Change," in Committee on Food Habits, *The Problem of Changing Food Habits: Report of the Committee on Food Habits 1941–1943*, Bulletin of the National Research Council No. 108 (October 1943), 35–65.

66. Bentley, *Eating for Victory*, 9–14; Lewis A. Erenberg and Susan E. Hirsch, eds., *The War in American Culture: Society and Consciousness during World War II* (Chicago: University of Chicago Press, 1996), 2–7.

67. Bentley, *Eating for Victory*, 11.

68. Erenberg and Hirsch, *The War in American Culture*, 5.

69. Robert Crawford, "The Boundaries of the Self and the Unhealthy Other: Reflections on Health, Culture and AIDS," *Social Science Medicine* 38, no. 10 (1994).

70. Alan Brinkley, *The End of Reform* (New York: Alfred A. Knopf, 1995), 202.

71. Brinkley, *The End of Reform*, 210–11, 213. Union membership rose from 3 million in 1933 to 8.5 million in 1940.

72. International Labour Office, *Nutrition in Industry* (Montreal: International Labour Office, 1946), 47.

73. *Proceedings of the National Nutrition Conference for Defense*, 128.

74. Committee on Nutrition in Industry, National Research Council, *The Food and Nutrition of Industrial Workers in Wartime* (Washington, DC: National Research Council, 1942).

75. *Proceedings of the National Nutrition Conference for Defense*, 127.

76. Committee on Nutrition in Industry, National Research Council, *The Food and Nutrition of Industrial Workers in Wartime*. The Committee on Nutrition in Industry was later renamed the Committee on Nutrition of Industrial Workers.

77. Division of Campaigns, Office of War Information, in Cooperation with Nutrition Division of Health and Welfare Services, *Better Health: A Speedier Victory through Proper Nutrition*, book 6 of the U.S. Government Campaign to Promote the Production, Sharing and Proper Use of Food (Washington, DC: U.S. Government Printing Office, 1943).

78. Robert Goodhart, "Wartime Feeding of Industrial Workers," in *Nutrition and the Food Supply: The War and After*, ed. John D. Black, vol. 225 of *Annals of the American Academy of Political and Social Science* (Philadelphia: American Academy of Political and Social Science, 1943), 118. "Better Nutrition Sought by McNutt," *New York Times*, August 10, 1942.

79. "Better Nutrition Sought by McNutt."

80. "Better Nutrition Sought by McNutt."

81. U.S. Department of Agriculture, War Food Administration, Nutrition and Food Conservation Branch, *Manual of Industrial Nutrition* (Washington, DC: U.S. Government Printing Office, 1943).

82. Seven regional industrial representatives advised plant executives on improving in-plant feeding conditions and setting up nutrition-education programs for employees. They also provided information about available posters, pamphlets, flyers, news releases, and programs, and suggested nutritionally sound menus that were compatible with food shortages and the rationing program. Ibid.

83. U.S. Department of Agriculture, *Manual of Industrial Nutrition.*

84. International Labour Office, *Nutrition in Industry*, 48.

85. U.S. Department of Agriculture, Bureau of Agricultural Economics, *Nutrition and the War: Opinions about Food, and Their Significance for Better Nutrition* (Washington, DC: U.S. Government Printing Office, 1943), 13.

86. U.S. Department of Agriculture, *Nutrition and the War*, 26–27.

87. U.S. Department of Agriculture, *Nutrition and the War*, 27.

88. Committee on Nutrition of Industrial Workers, Food and Nutrition Board, *Nutrition of Industrial Workers*, second report of the Committee on Nutrition of Industrial Workers (Washington, DC: National Research Council, 1945), 13–14.

89. Anderson, *Wartime Women*, 4.

90. Perry R. Duis, "No Time for Privacy: World War II and Chicago's Families," in *The War in American Culture: Society and Consciousness during World War II*, ed. Lewis A. Erenberg and Susan E. Hirsch (Chicago: University of Chicago Press, 1996); Anderson, *Wartime Women.*

91. "First Lady Appeals for Unified People," *New York Times*, November 18, 1941.

92. "We Eat to Work," Cornell University radio brief, *Everyday Living in Wartime* series, 6 January 1944.

93. "Better Nutrition Sought by McNutt," *New York Times*, August 10, 1942.

94. Kurt Lewin, "Forces Behind Food Habits and Methods of Change."

95. U.S. Department of Agriculture, Bureau of Agricultural Economics, *Nutrition and the War*, 10.

96. U.S. Department of Agriculture, *Nutrition and the War*, 11.

97. "Kitchen Kommando," Ithaca: New York State College of Home Economics, Department of Food and Nutrition, "Records #23–2–749."

98. Ted Jung, United States War Food Administration, *For Work, for Play, 3 'Squares' a Day: Eat the Basic 7 Way* (Washington, DC: U.S. Government Printing Office, 1944).

99. Consumer Counsel Division of the U.S. Department of Agriculture, "Mrs. America Volunteers," special issue, *Consumer's Guide* 7, no. 20 (October 15, 1941), 2–3.

100. Gyorgy Scrinis, "Sorry, Marge," *Meanjin* 61, no. 4 (2002).

FOUR
From Microscopes to "Macroscopes"

1. On "macroscopes," see Joan Dye Gussow, "Growth, Truth, and Responsibility: Food Is the Bottom Line," Occasional Paper Series, 2, no. 6 (Greensboro: Institute of Nutrition, University of North Carolina, 1981). Gussow was the author of the classic *The Feeding Web: Issues in Nutritional Ecology* (Palo Alto, CA: Bull Publishing, 1978).

2. Gussow, "Growth, Truth, and Responsibility," 4, 10.

3. Julie Guthman uses "alternative food" to refer to "institutions and practices that bring small-scale farmers, artisan food producers, and restaurant chefs together with consumers for the market exchange of what is characterized as fresh, local, seasonal organic, craft produced food." Julie Guthman, *Weighing In*, 3. Using a broader interpretation, Rachel Slocum identifies four broad types of alternative-food projects. Some organizations supported local farmers, promoting farmers markets, community-supported agriculture, buy-local campaigns, and changes in agricultural policies. At the same time, environmentally focused activists promoted organic, free-range, and hormone- and antibiotic-free meats as well as the protection of agricultural diversity and culinary heritage. Another group of organizations were concerned primarily with social justice, with some focusing on workers' rights and others on issues related to food insecurity. Slocum also includes nonprofit groups that focused their efforts on nutrition education, cooking demonstrations, and obesity prevention. Rachel Slocum, "Whiteness, Space and Alternative Food Practice," *Geoform* 38 (2007), 522.

4. Alice Julier, for example, warns against characterizing this as a "movement" in the singular, "led by some white men writing books, giving talks, and providing 'rules' for eating, and some women telling you that the kitchen and the farm are now free of the oppressive qualities that made a commercial food system and unequal treatment in the paid labor force more attractive than servitude or housework." Alice Julier, "How Not to Define Your Social Movement: Notes on Feminism, Intersectionality, and Food," paper presented at the "Food Networks: Gender and Foodways" conference, University of Notre Dame Gender Studies Program, Notre Dame, Indiana, January 26–28, 2012.

5. Julie Guthman, *Agrarian Dreams: The Paradox of Organic Farming in California* (Berkeley: University of California Press, 2004), 3–7.

6. Warren Belasco, *Appetite for Change: How the Counter Culture Took on the Food Industry, 1966–1988* (Ithaca, NY: Cornell University Press, 1989), 22–36, 44.

7. Wendell Berry, "Land Use," in *Last Whole Earth Catalog* (June 1971), 46. See also Guthman, *Agrarian Dreams*.

8. Wendell Berry, "Agricultural Solutions for Agricultural Problems," in *Bringing It to the Table: On Farming and Food* (Berkeley: Counterpoint, 2009), 29.

9. Frances Moore Lappé, *Diet for a Small Planet* (New York: Ballantine, 1971).

10. Joan Dye Gussow, "PCBs For Breakfast and Other Problems of a Food System Gone Awry," *Food Monitor* (May–June 1982), 26.

11. Guthman, *Agrarian Dreams*, chap. 2.

12. Guthman, *Agrarian Dreams*, chap. 2.

13. Eric Schlosser, *Fast Food Nation: The Dark Side of the All-American Meal* (Boston: Houghton Mifflin, 2001).

14. Marion Nestle, *Food Politics: How the Food Industry Influences Nutrition and Health* (Berkeley: University of California Press, 2002).

15. Charlotte Biltekoff, "Functional Foods for Health: Negotiation and Implications," NABC Report 22, *Promoting Health by Linking Agriculture, Food, and Nutrition: Proceedings of the twenty-second annual conference of the National Agricultural Biotechnology Council*, University of California, Davis, June 16–18, 2010, ed. Allan Eaglesham, Alan B. Bennet, and Ralph W. F. Hardy (Ithaca, NY: National Agricultural Biotechnology Council, 2010), 99–108; Clare Hasler, "The Changing Face of Functional Foods," *Journal of the American College of Nutrition* 19, no. 5 (2000); Mark Lawrence and Mike Rayner, "Functional Foods and Health Claims: A Public Health Policy Perspective," *Public Health Nutrition* 1, no. 2 (1998).

16. Holuigue, Dianne. "Alice's Wonderland." *Epicurean*, September 1988.

17. Alice Waters, "The Farm-Restaurant Connection," in *Our Sustainable Table*, ed. Robert Clark (San Francisco: North Point Press, 1990), 114.

18. Alice Waters, Linda P. Guenzel, and Carolyn Dille, *The Chez Panisse Menu Cookbook*, 1st edn. (New York: Random House, 1982), 2.

19. Seven Chez Panisse cookbooks have been published, several of which include forewords or prefaces by Waters in which she explains her ethos and ideals. Waters is author or coauthor of all but one of the books, and has also published two additional cookbooks, a children's book, and a Chez Panisse fortieth anniversary tribute collection, which advance her ideals but are not directly related to the Chez Panisse kitchen.

20. Michael Pollan, *The Omnivore's Dilemma: A Natural History of Four Meals* (New York: Penguin, 2006), 7.

21. Michael Pollan, *In Defense of Food: An Eater's Manifesto* (New York: Penguin, 2008).

22. Waters cites and expands on Berry's "Pleasures of the Table," in Alice Waters, "The Delicious Revolution," paper presented at the Environmental Grantmakers Association 1999 Retreat, Pacific Grove, California, October 25, 1999; and Alice Waters, Alan Tangren, and Fritz Streiff, *Chez Panisse Fruit* (New York: HarperCollins, 2002), xvi. Pollan expands on Berry in his introduction to Wendell Berry, *Bringing It to the Table: On Farming and Food* (Berkeley: Counterpoint, 2009), x; and Pollan, *In Defense of Food*, 161.

23. Wendell Berry, "The Pleasure of Eating," in *Bringing It to the Table: On Farming and Food* (Berkeley: Counterpoint, 2009), 233–34.

24. Waters, Tangren, and Streiff, *Chez Panisse Fruit*, xvi.

25. Fixed-price meals are still served nightly at Chez Panisse. Since 1980 the Chez Panisse Café has served an à la carte menu upstairs from the restaurant.

26. Linda Witt, "Stirring Up a Cooking Revolution," *Chicago Tribune Sunday Magazine*, May 11, 1986.

27. Pollan, *The Omnivore's Dilemma*, 11.

28. Pollan, *The Omnivore's Dilemma*, 142–44.

29. Pollan, *In Defense of Food*, 12.

30. Michael Pollan, *Food Rules: An Eater's Manifesto* (New York: Penguin, 2009); Michael Pollan and Maira Kalman, *Food Rules: An Eater's Manual* (New York: Penguin, 2011).

31. Guthman writes, "Thanks to its confluence with the neoliberal economic project, healthism morphed from a critical perspective on both the biomedical establishment and industrial toxins, to an embrace of self-care, to an utter devolution of health responsibility to the individual in the interest of both reducing the health care costs of the body politic and performing fitness"; Guthman, *Weighing In*, 56.

32. Robert Crawford, "Health as Meaningful Social Practice," *Health* 10, no. 4 (2006), 408.

33. Crawford, "Health as Meaningful Social Practice," 402.

34. For more on healthism, see Robert Crawford, "Healthism and the Medicalization of Everyday Life," *International Journal of Health Services* 10, no. 3 (1980); and Guthman, *Weighing In*.

35. Nestle, *Food Politics*, 39.

36. Guthman, *Weighing In*, 17–18.

37. Joan Dye Gussow, *This Organic Life: Confessions of a Surburban Homesteader* (White River Junction, VT: Chelsea Green Publishing, 2001), 175, 215.

38. Barbara Kingsolver, Steven L. Hopp, and Camille Kingsolver, *Animal, Vegetable, Miracle: A Year of Food Life* (New York: HarperCollins, 2007), 22.

39. Pollan, *The Omnivore's Dilemma*, 9.

40. J. Peck and A. Tickell, "Neoliberalizing Space," *Antipode* 43, no. 3 (2002).

41. Peck and Tickell, "Neoliberalizing Space"; David Harvey, *A Brief History of Neoliberalism* (New York: Oxford University Press, 2005). Mary Beth Pudop describes these projects as "voluntary and third sector initiatives organized around principles of self-improvement and moral responsibility [that] stand in for state sponsored social policies and programs premised on collective responses to social risk." Mary Beth Pudup, "It Takes a Garden: Cultivating Citizen-Subjects in Organized Garden Projects," *Geoforum* 39, no. 3 (2008), 1229.

42. Guthman, Julie. "Neoliberalism and the Making of Food Politics in California." *Geoforum* 39, no. 3 (2008). Guthman and Allen argue, for example, that while many alternative food activists were opposed to the displacement of state governance to private and international organizations, "the populist localism they do embrace

happens to resonate with the neoliberal devolution of responsibility and accountability to the local." Julie Guthman and Patricia Allen, "From 'Old School' to 'Farm-to-School': Neoliberalism from the Ground Up," *Agriculture and Human Values* 23 (2006), 409.

43. Thomas McNamee, *Alice Waters and Chez Panisse* (New York: Penguin, 2007), 204.

44. Waters, "Slow Food, Slow Schools: Teaching Sustainability through the Education of the Senses," paper presented at the program in agrarian studies at Yale University, New Haven, Connecticut, 2003.

45. Charles Burres, "The Delicious Revolution Honored," *San Francisco Chronicle*, August 4, 1998.

46. The Chez Panisse Foundation was inaugurated under Waters's leadership in August 1996, on the occasion of the restaurant's twenty-fifth anniversary. By the end of that year, $39,000 had been raised under its auspices, and annual income consistently increased, from $151,000 in 1997 to nearly $400,000 in 2002. Marjorie Rice, "Chefs: War and Peas," *San Francisco Examiner*, December 30, 1992.

47. "Our Founding Programs," Edible Schoolyard Project website, available at http://edibleschoolyard.org/node/95.

48. Waters, "Slow Food, Slow Schools: Teaching Sustainability through the Education of the Senses," 1.

49. Ellen Richards, "Social Significance of the Home Economics Movement," *Journal of Home Economics* 3, no. 2 (1911), 118, 122.

50. Richards, "Social Significance of the Home Economics Movement," 118, 122. See also Alice Waters, "The Ethics of Eating: Part Two," paper presented at the Sixteenth Annual Ecological Farming Conference, Asilomar, California, January 25, 1996; Alice Waters, "A Letter to Clinton and Gore," December 9, 1995, *EarthLight*, available at http://www.earthlight.org/alicewaters23.html.

51. Ellen Richards, "Luncheons for School," *New England Kitchen*, May 1895, 51.

52. Ellen Richards, "Social Significance of the Home Economics Movement," 118, 122. Like Waters, some home economists also suggested using "lunch as a syllabus" and urged schools to pay attention to "ethics, table manners and conversation." Ira S. Wile, "School Lunches," *Journal of Home Economics* (1910), 168, 163.

53. Elizabeth Crane, "The Incredible, Edible Schoolyard," *District Administration*, July 2003, available at http://www.districtadministration.com/article/incredible-edible-schoolyard.

54. Zilah Bahar, "Personal Taste: Many Lessons Are Taught at the Edible Schoolyard," *San Francisco Examiner*, August 18, 1999.

55. Alice Waters, "December 17 Letter to Bill Clinton," Chez Panisse, Inc. records, BANC MSS 2001/148 c, Bancroft Library, University of California, Berkeley, 1996.

56. Writing about the Edible Schoolyard, Mary Beth Pudup points out that while the curriculum encompassed both production and consumption "*the real action is in the kitchen* . . . where consumer subjects are produced around cooking and eating." Pudup, "It Takes a Garden," 1238.

57. Guthman and Allen, "From 'Old School' to 'Farm-to-School,'" 411–12.

58. Deborah Lupton and Alan Petersen, *The New Public Health: Health and Self in the Age of Risk* (London: Sage, 1996), 95.

59. Robert Crawford, "The Boundaries of the Self and the Unhealthy Other: Reflections on Health, Culture and AIDS," *Social Science Medicine* 38, no. 10 (1994), 1352.

60. Belasco, *Appetite for Change*, 194.

61. Belasco, *Appetite for Change*, 196–97.

62. Pollan, *In Defense of Food*, 187. Also see Colin McEnroe, "A Thoughtful, Simple Menu," *Hartford Courant*, January 3, 2008.

63. Pollan, *In Defense of Food*, 187.

64. Pollan, *In Defense of Food*, 187.

65. Alice Waters, "Speech to the Baker's Guild," paper presented at the REAP Conference, Madison, Wisconsin, September 1998, 3.

66. Alice Waters, "Fast Food Values," keynote address at REAP conference, Madison, Wisconsin, September 2002. See also Paul Rauber, "Conservation a la Carte," *Sierra*, November–December 1994.

67. Waters, "Fast Food Values," 2.

68. Alics Waters, "The Ethics of Eating," paper presented at the Mills College Commencement, Oakland, California, May 22, 1994.

69. Laura Shapiro, "The War on Alice Waters," *Gourmet*, May 6, 2009, available at http://www.gourmet.com/foodpolitics/2009/05/war-on-alice-waters.

70. Rauber, "Conservation à la Carte"; Ken Kelley, "Alice Waters," *Mother Jones*, January–February 1995, available at http://www.motherjones.com/politics/1995/01/alice-waters; "Alice's Restaurant," *Cooks Magazine*, January/February, 1983; "Nurturing Connections with Farmers: An Interview with Alice Waters," *In Season: A Report on Locally Grown Produce*, 1997, available at http://marketreport.com/waters.htm.

71. "Alice Waters' Crusade for Better Food," *60 Minutes*, CBS, March 15, 2009.

72. A selected sample of blogs that discussed and debated charges of elitism in response to this segment: Alison Stein Wellner, "Waters-gate? Alice Waters' Controversial Role in the Obama Vegetable Garden," March 20, 2009, available at http://www.huffingtonpost.com/alison-stein-wellner/waters-gate-alice-waters_b_177358.html; Eat Me Daily, "Alice Water's Political Flailings: A Misguided Love Story," March 2, 2009, available at http://www.eatmedaily.com/2009/03/alice-waters-political-flailings-a-misguided-love-story/.

73. "Alice Waters' Crusade for Better Food."

74. Michael Pollan, "Why Eating Well Is 'Elitist,'" *New York Times* "On the Table Blog," May 11, 2006. http://michaelpollan.com/articles-archive/why-eating-well-is-elitist/.

75. Ian Brown, "Author Michael Pollan Explains the War on Food Movement," *Globe and Mail*, March 18, 2011, available at http://www.theglobeandmail.com/life/author-michael-pollan-explains-the-war-on-food-movement/article573363.

76. Crawford, "The Boundaries of the Self and the Unhealthy Other," 1356.

77. Lappé, "Food, Farming and Democracy," 150.

78. Kingsolver, Hopp, and Kingsolver, *Animal, Vegetable, Miracle*, 127.

79. Kingsolver, Hopp, and Kingsolver, *Animal, Vegetable, Miracle*, 130.

80. Weingarten, "Alice's Wonderland." *Newsweek*, August 27, 2001, 45.

81. Waters, "Fast Food Values," 2.

82. Waters, "Slow Food, Slow Schools: Teaching Sustainability through the Education of the Senses"; Waters, "Fast Food Values."

83. Susan Ives, "Feeding Hearts and Minds: Interview: Alice Waters," *Land and People*, November 7, 2000, available at http://www.tpl.org/publications/land-and-people-magazine/archive/landpeople-fall-1999/feeding-hearts-and-minds.html.

84. Tara Weingarten, "Alice's Wonderland," *Newsweek*, August 27, 2001.

85. Waters, "The Ethics of Eating," 5.

86. Waters, "The Ethics of Eating," 5.

87. Waters, "Fast Food Values," 4.

88. Deborah Lupton, *Food, the Body and the Self* (London: Sage, 1996), 87–88.

89. Julie Guthman argues that this opposition elides the reality that the growth of "slow food" was driven by many of the same historical and economic factors that led to growth of fast food. She points out that organic production depended on "the same system of marginal labor as [did] fast food," that "organic salad mix led the way in convenience packaging and [was] often grown out of place and out of season," and that "many of those who [ate] organic food came into their wealth from some of the very processes that enabled the fast food industry's growth." While materially false, the presumed binary opposition between fast and slow food was ideologically powerful. As Guthman argues, it imparted "a good deal of subjectivity onto the organic or slow food eater while the fast food eater [was] treated as a mindless dupe." Julie Guthman, "Fast Food/Organic Food: Reflexive Tastes and the Making of 'Yuppie Chow,'" *Social and Cultural Geography* 4, no. 1 (2003), 46, 55.

90. Alice Waters, "Slow Food, Slow Schools: Transforming Education through a School Lunch Curriculum," a speech by Alice Waters, October 2003, available at www.edibleschoolyard.org/Alice_message.html.

91. Pollan, *In Defense of Food*, 168, 170, 187.

92. Waters, "The Ethics of Eating: Part Two," 5.

93. Kelley, "Alice Waters."

94. Witt, "Stirring Up a Cooking Revolution"; Waters, "Slow Food, Slow Schools: Teaching Sustainability through the Education of the Senses"; Waters, "Slow Food, Slow Schools: Transforming Education through a School Lunch Curriculum."

95. Waters, "Slow Food, Slow Schools," 10.

96. Pollan, *In Defense of Food*, 13.

97. Waters, "The Ethics of Eating," 1.

98. Waters, "The Farm-Restaurant Connection," 115.

FIVE
Thinness as Health, Self-Control, and Citizenship

1. Megan Mulligan, "Michelle Obama to Create an Organic 'Victory' Garden at the White House," *Guardian* (March 20, 2009), available at http://www.guardiannews.com.

2. Kate Barret and Brian Hartman, "Foodies Celebrate White House Veggie Garden," *ABC News* (March 20, 2009), available at http://abcnews.go.com/Health/story?id=7110660&page=1; Darlene Superville, "Ground Is Broken for White House 'Kitchen Garden,'" *SFGate* (March 20, 2009), available at http://www.sfgate.com.

3. "Remarks by the First Lady at the White House Garden Harvest Party," White House Office of the First Lady (June 16, 2009), available at http://www.whitehouse.gov/the-press-office/remarks-first-lady-white-house-garden-harvest-party.

4. Marian Burros, "Obamas to Plant a Vegetable Garden at the White House," *New York Times*, March 20, 2009.

5. "Remarks by the First Lady at the White House Garden Harvest Party."

6. For astute analysis at this intersection, see Julie Guthman, "Can't Stomach It: How Michael Pollan et al. Made Me Want to Eat Cheetos," *Gastronomica* (summer 2007); Julie Guthman, "Fast Food/Organic Food: Reflexive Tastes and the Making of 'Yuppie Chow,'" *Social and Cultural Geography* 4, no. 1 (2003); Julie Guthman, *Weighing In: Obesity, Food Justice, and the Limits of Capitalism* (Berkeley: University of California, 2011).

7. Peggy Orenstein, "Food Fighter," *New York Times Magazine*, March 7, 2004, available at http://www.nytimes.com/2004/03/07/magazine/food-fighter.html?pagewanted=all&src=pm.

8. Michael Pollan, "The Way We Live Now: The (Agri)Cultural Contradictions of Obesity," *New York Times Magazine*, October 12, 2003, available at http://www.nytimes.com/2003/10/12/magazine/12WWLN.html?pagewanted=all; Michael Pollan, *In Defense of Food: An Eater's Manifesto* (New York: Penguin, 2008).

9. Marilyn Wann, "Fat Studies: An Invitation to Revolution," in *The Fat Studies Reader*, ed. Sondra Solovay and Esther Rothblum (New York: NYU Press, 2009), xiii; Julie Guthman, "Neoliberalism and the Constitution of Contemporary Bodies," in *The Fat Studies Reader*, 188.

10. Eric J. Oliver, *Fat Politics: The Real Story behind America's Obesity Epidemic* (New York: Oxford University Press, 2006), 47–49.

11. Marketdata Enterprise, press release from PR Web, May 9, 2011, accessed February 15, 2013, available at http://www.prweb.com/releases/2011/5/prweb8393658.htm.

12. Pat Lyons, "Prescription for Harm: Diet Industry Influence, Public Health, and the 'Obesity Epidemic,'" in Solovay and Rothblum, *The Fat Studies Reader*, 75.

13. Abigail C. Saguy and Kevin W. Riley, "Weighing Both Sides: Morality, Mortality, and Framing Contests over Obesity," *Journal of Health Politics, Policy and Law* 30, no. 5 (2005), 869.

14. Saguy and Riley, "Weighing Both Sides," 875–77.

15. Saguy and Riley, "Weighing Both Sides," 875–77.

16. For a discussion of the nineteenth-century roots of moral and aesthetic concerns about obesity, see Amy Erdman Farrell, *Fat Shame: Stigma and the Fat Body in American Culture* (New York: NYU Press, 2011). Peter Stearns describes the postwar intensification of moral and aesthetic concerns, as well as the emergence of medical concerns about the relationship between fatness and health, in *Fat History: Bodies and Beauty in the Modern West* (New York: NYU Press, 1997), chaps. 1 and 2.

17. Roberta Pollack Seid, *Never Too Thin: Why Women Are at War with Their Bodies* (New York: Prentice Hall, 1989), 116.

18. Seid, *Never Too Thin*, 118.

19. "Overeating Called 'Compulsive': Diet Held Only Way to Reduce," *New York Times*, October 21, 1950.

20. "Eating Less Urged for Those over 25: Obesity a National Malady," *New York Times*, April 17, 1952; Howard A. Rusk, "Overweight Persons Termed Top Health Problem in U.S.," *New York Times*, April 17, 1952.

21. "Overeating Laid to U.S.," *New York Times*, April 4, 1950.

22. "Overeating Called 'Compulsive.'"

23. Stearns, *Fat History*, 11.

24. Seid, *Never Too Thin*, 139.

25. David Mark Hegsted, "Recollections of a Pioneer in Nutrition: Fifty Years in Nutrition," *Journal of the College of Nutrition* 9, no. 4 (1990).

26. Patricia Crotty, *Good Nutrition?: Fact and Fashion in Dietary Advice* (St. Leonards, Australia: Allen and Unwin, 1995), 53.

27. Seid, *Never Too Thin*, 141.

28. Marion Nestle, *Food Politics: How the Food Industry Influences Nutrition and Health* (Berkeley: University of California Press, 2002), 39.

29. Nestle, *Food Politics*.

30. The advice infuriated the major food producers, who feared that consumers would turn away from their products and mounted a major offensive against the guidelines. For more on the controversy, see Nestle, *Food Politics*, 38–50. Conversely, fat as a focus for negative nutrition did not anger food interests as much and actually opened new commercial opportunities. Levenstein points out that this may have caused experts to be less ready to challenge "some of the questionable 'facts' on which it was based." Harvey Levenstein, *Paradox of Plenty: A Social History of Eating in Modern America* (New York: Oxford University Press, 1993), 241.

31. Nestle, *Food Politics*, 40.

32. Stearns, *Fat History*, 111, 14.

33. Stearns, *Fat History*, 125.

34. William H. Dietz, Barbara Browman, James S. Marks, and Jeffrey P. Koplan, "The Spread of the Obesity Epidemic in the United States," *Journal of the American Medical Association* 282, no. 16 (October 1999).

35. Paul Campos, *The Obesity Myth: Why America's Obsession with Weight Is Hazardous to Your Health* (New York: Gotham Books, 2004); Katherine M. Flegal and R. J. Kuczymarski, "Criteria for Definition of Overweight in Transition: Background and Recommendations for the United States," *American Journal of Clinical Nutrition* 72 (2000); Nanci Hellmich, "Fat Is in Your BMI, but Also in the Eye of the Beholder," *USA Today*, June 10, 1998. In another argument questioning the data that spurred the declaration of an obesity epidemic, Jeffrey Friedman, an obesity researcher at Rockefeller University, pointed out that national data did not indicate that Americans were growing uniformly fatter. In the midrange there had been an increase of about six or seven

pounds between 1991 and 2004. More people crossed the line from normal to obese, but the average weight of the population increased only seven to ten pounds. Gina Kolata, "The Fat Epidemic: He Says It's an Illusion," *New York Times*, June 8, 2004.

36. Oliver, *Fat Politics*, 18–19.

37. See Julie Guthman's *Weighing In*, chap. 2, for an in-depth discussion and critique of the BMI as a measure of both adiposity and health. Of particular relevance to my discussion, Guthman writes, "The use of the BMI has redefined obesity away from being a question of impaired functionality and toward one of form." Guthman, *Weighing In*, 29; see also chap. 2.

38. Guthman challenges the energy balance model (too many calories consumed, too few expended) and makes a compelling case for epigenetic causes of obesity, including exposures to chemicals and food substances. See *Weighing In*, chap. 5.

39. Bharathi Radhakrishnan, "Can Air Conditioning Make You Fat?," June 27, 2006. ABC News Online, available at http://abcnews.go.com/Health/Diet/story?id=2120381&page=1.

40. Michael Singer, "Fat of the Land," *New York Times Magazine*, April 3, 2001.

41. Farrell, *Fat Shame*, 64.

42. Stearns, *Fat History*, 54–65.

43. Stearns, *Fat History*, 5, 126.

44. Kathleen LeBesco, "Neoliberalism, Public Health, and the Moral Perils of Fatness," *Critical Public Health* (2010), 2.

45. Robert Crawford, "A Cultural Account of 'Health': Control, Release, and the Social Body," in *Issues on the Political Economy of Health Care*, ed. John B. McKinley (New York: Tavistock, 1984), 70. Kathleen LeBesco also describes the growing conflation of body size, health, and morality: "Fatness seems to equate instantaneously with unhealthiness, and thinness with healthiness, based on a false presumption about the transparency of these bodies in terms of the actions they undertake." LeBesco, "Neoliberalism, Public Health, and the Moral Perils of Fatness," 3; see also Kathleen LeBesco, *Revolting Bodies?: The Struggle to Redefine Fat Identity* (Amherst: University of Massachusetts Press, 2004).

46. Campos, *The Obesity Myth*, 142. The study was conducted by Campos for the book, which was published in 2004.

47. The purpose of the Harvard study was to examine whether obese patients value modest reductions in weight. The researchers asked this question in response to prior studies showing that weight-loss patients often had unrealistic weight-loss goals and were disappointed when they did not meet their goals. The subjects were asked about what they would be willing to risk or give up to be a certain weight, an established approach used to quantify the quality of life of people living with different diseases. The technique was adapted to describe the preferences that primary-care patients have for different levels of weight and weight loss, specifically modest weight loss. Christina C. Wee, Mary B. Hamel, Roger B. Davis, and Russell S. Phillips, "Assessing the Value of Weight Loss among Primary Care Patients," *Journal of General Internal Medicine* 19 (2004); Gina Kolata, "Longing to Lose, at a Cost," *New York Times*, January 4, 2005.

48. Sondra Solovay, *Tipping the Scales of Justice: Fighting Weight-Based Discrimination* (Amherst, NY: Prometheus Books, 2000), 25.

49. Crotty, *Good Nutrition?*, 66–71.

50. Oliver, *Fat Politics*, 38–43.

51. Oliver, *Fat Politics*, 38–43.

52. Oliver, *Fat Politics*, 42. Oliver reframes the obesity epidemic as an epidemic of *ideas*, and traces its emergence and viruslike spread to Dietz, who he refers to as "patient zero." See Oliver, 38–43, for a comprehensive overview of the role Dietz's slides played in the formation of what would become known as the obesity epidemic.

53. Saguy and Riley, "Weighing Both Sides," 892.

54. Saguy and Riley, "Weighing Both Sides," 892. See also Michael Fumento, "Obesity Is Contagious," *American Spectator*, August 1, 2007, available at http://spectator.org/archives/2007/08/01/obesity-is-contagious.

55. Saguy and Riley, "Weighing Both Sides," 875–76; Oliver, *Fat Politics*, 36.

56. U.S. Department of Health and Human Services, *The Surgeon General's Call to Action to Prevent and Decrease Overweight and Obesity* (Rockland, MD: U.S. Department of Health and Human Services, Public Health Service, Office of the Surgeon General, 2001).

57. Crawford, "A Cultural Account of 'Health,'" 76–77."

58. LeBesco, "Neoliberalism, Public Health, and the Moral Perils of Fatness"; Deborah Lupton and Alan Petersen, *The New Public Health: Health and Self in the Age of Risk* (London: Sage, 1996); Guthman, "Neoliberalism and the Constitution of Contemporary Bodies."

59. Guthman, "Neoliberalism and the Constitution of Contemporary Bodies," 193.

60. Crawford argues, "Individual responsibility for health, although not without challenge, proved to be particularly effective in establishing the 'common sense' of neoliberalism's essential tenets." Robert Crawford, "Health as Meaningful Social Practice," *Health* 10, no. 4 (2006).

61. Roniece Weaver, Fabiola D. Gaines, and Angela Ebron, *Slim Down Sister: The African American Woman's Guide to Healthy, Permanent Weight Loss* (New York: Dutton, 2000), 6.

62. Atul Gawande, "The Man Who Couldn't Stop Eating," *New Yorker*, July 9, 2001, 71.

63. Jane Clemen, Diana Kirkwood, Bobbi Schell, and Daniel Myerson, *The Town that Lost a Ton: How One Town Used the Buddy System to Lose 3,998 Pounds . . . and How You Can Too!* (Naperville, IL: Sourcebooks, 2002), 49, 154.

64. LeBesco, "Neoliberalism, Public Health, and the Moral Perils of Fatness," 194, citing Alan Petersen, "Governmentality, Critical Scholarship, and the Medical Humanities," *Journal of Medical Humanities*, 24, no. 3/4 (winter 2003), 187–201.

65. George W. Bush, "Remarks by the President on Fitness," Lakewest Family YMCA, Dallas, Texas, July 18, 2003, available at http://www.whitehouse.gov/news/releases/2003/07/20030718–6.html.

66. Julie Guthman, "Neoliberalism and the Making of Food Politics in California"; LeBesco, "Neoliberalism, Public Health, and the Moral Perils of Fatness."

67. Guthman, *Weighing In*, 66. See *Weighing In*, chap. 4, "Does Your Neighborhood Make You Fat?" for an in-depth analysis and critique of the theory that obesity is caused by particular built environments.

68. Kelly D. Brownell and Katherine Battle Horgen, *Food Fight: The Inside Story of the Food Industry, America's Obesity Crisis, and What We Can Do About It* (New York: McGraw-Hill, 2004), 5.

69. Brownell and Horgen, *Food Fight*, 309–13.

70. Michael Pollan, *The Omnivore's Dilemma: A Natural History of Four Meals* (New York: Penguin, 2006), 107.

71. Pollan, *The Omnivore's Dilemma*, 102.

72. Pollan, *In Defense of Food*, 10. See Guthman, *Weighing In*, chap. 6, "Does Farm Policy Make You Fat?" for an in-depth analysis and critique of these claims.

73. Guthman, "Neoliberalism and the Constitution of Contemporary Bodies," 188–89. See also Saguy and Riley, "Weighing Both Sides," 888. Guthman argues that the obesogenic-environment thesis produces a false equivalence between environmental factors and obesity rates only by ignoring the class and racial aspects of those environments, and erroneously assuming that differences in body size accrue to the built environment itself independent of who can, wants to, and does live in those environments. Guthman, *Weighing In*, chap. 4.

74. Taeku Lee and Eric J. Oliver, "Public Opinion and the Politics of America's Obesity Epidemic," Social Science Research Network, May 2002, available at http://papers.ssrn.com/so13/papers.cfm?abstract_id=313824.

75. Samantha Kwan, "Individual Versus Corporate Responsibility," *Food, Culture and Society* 12, no. 4 (2009), 483, 486, 488.

76. Kwan, "Individual Versus Corporate Responsibility," 490.

77. For more on the following arguments about the relationship between the war on obesity and the War on Terror see Biltekoff, "The Terror Within: Obesity in Post 9/11 U.S. Life."

78. Oliver, *Fat Politics*, 37; Saguy and Riley, "Weighing Both Sides," 875–76.

79. Greg Critser, *Fat Land: How Americans Became the Fattest People in the World* (Boston: Houghton Mifflin, 2003), 170.

80. U.S. Department of Health and Human Services, *The Surgeon General's Call to Action to Prevent and Decrease Overweight and Obesity*.

81. Reuters, "U.S. Male Soldiers Are Getting Fatter," *San Diego Union-Tribune*, November 10, 2001.

82. Lisa Hoffman, "Half of U.S. Military Population Overweight, Study Says: A Few Extra Pounds Likely to Affect Combat Readiness of a Few Good Men," *Washington Times*, January 1, 2002.

83. Hoffman, "Half of U.S. Military Population Overweight."

84. Robert A. Rosenblatt, "Surgeon General Takes Stern Stance on Obesity," *Los Angeles Times*, December 14, 2001.

85. Kim Severson, "Obesity 'a Threat' to U.S. Security: Surgeon General Urges Cultural Shift," *San Francisco Chronicle*, January 7, 2003; Melissa Healy, "War on Fat Gets Serious," *Los Angeles Times*, January 3, 2004.

86. Craig Lambert, "The Way We Eat Now: Ancient Bodies Collide with Modern Technology to Produce a Flabby, Disease-Ridden Populace," *Harvard Magazine*, May–June 2004.

87. "Interview with Surgeon General Richard Carmona," *Morning Edition*, National Public Radio, November 27, 2003.

88. Severson, "Obesity 'a Threat' to U.S. Security." See also "Surgeon General to Cops: Put Down the Donuts," CNN.com, March 2, 2003, available at http://www.cnn.com/2003/HEALTH/02/28/obesity.police.

89. Richard Carmona, "Remarks at the American Enterprise Institute Obesity Conference," U.S. Department of Health and Human Services, Washington, June 10, 2003, available at http://www.surgeongeneral.gov/news/speeches/obesity061003.html.

90. David L. Altheide, "Consuming Terrorism," *Symbolic Interaction* 27, no. 3 (2004).

91. George W. Bush, "Remarks by the President on Fitness," available at http://www.whitehouse.gov/news/releases/2003/07/20030718–6.html.

92. For a comprehensive look at terrorism and the politics of fear, see Altheide, "Consuming Terrorism"; David L. Altheide, *Terrorism and the Politics of Fear* (Lanham, MD: AltaMira Press, 2006).

93. Altheide, "Consuming Terrorism," 292.

94. Altheide, "Consuming Terrorism," 303.

95. Saguy and Riley, "Weighing Both Sides," 913.

96. Richard Carmona, "Remarks to the California Childhood Obesity Conference," U.S. Department of Health and Human Services, January 6, 2003, available at http://www.surgeongeneral.gov/news/speeches/califobesity.html.

97. Campos, *The Obesity Myth*, 17. The popularity of this figure as a warning and justification for antiobesity measures began with a misstatement of the findings of a 1993 *Journal of the American Medical Association* (JAMA) article by former Surgeon General C. Everett Koop. When warned about having misrepresented the JAMA findings by stating that obesity-related conditions "are the second leading cause of death in the U.S., resulting in about 300,000 lives lost each year," Koop is said to have defended his interpretation and claimed that it would eventually be verified. His interpretation, meanwhile, became the primary reference the Food and Drug Administration used in deciding that obesity was a disease that could be helped by drugs. In the spring of 2004 the CDC increased the number of yearly deaths attributable to obesity to 400,000 in a report coauthored by the agency's director. By the fall of that same year, however, the government began working on a rare correction after other CDC statisticians found serious errors in the calculations. By the spring of 2005, the figure faced its greatest crisis of authority yet, with the CDC reporting in JAMA that its figures had been grossly exaggerated due to methodological errors and reducing their estimate of annual deaths attributable to obesity to roughly 26,000. The same report also found that people who were somewhat overweight were less at risk of early death than people who were thin. See C. Everett Koop, "Dr. C. Everett Koop Launches a New 'Crusade' to Combat Obesity in America," Shape Up Amer-

ica!, December 6, 1994, available at http://www.shapeup.org/about/arch_pr/120694.php; Laura Johaness and Steve Stecklow, "Dire Warnings about Obesity Rely on Slippery Statistics," *Wall Street Journal*, February 9, 1998; Katherine M. Flegal, David Williamson, Elsie Pamuk, and Harry M. Rosenberg, "Estimating Deaths Attributable to Obesity in the United States," *American Journal of Public Health* 94, no. 9 (September 2004); Katherine M. Flegal, Barry I. Graubard, David F. Williamson, and Mitchell H. Gail, "Excess Deaths Associated with Underweight, Overweight, and Obesity," *Journal of the American Medical Association* 293, no. 15 (2005).

98. Carmona, "Remarks to the California Childhood Obesity Conference."

99. Derrick Z. Jackson, "All Quiet on the Fat Front," *Boston Globe*, October 11, 2002.

100. Altheide, "Consuming Terrorism." See also Altheide, *Terrorism and the Politics of Fear*; Charlotte Biltekoff, "The Terror Within: Obesity in Post 9/11 U.S. Life," *American Studies* 48, no. 3 (2007).

101. A study comparing attitudes toward obesity in six nations determined that prejudice increased in individualist cultures, such as in the United States, where there was a tendency to hold people responsible for their obesity. Christian S. Crandall et al., "An Attribution-Value Model of Prejudice: Anti-Fat Attitudes in Six Nations," *Personality and Social Psychology Bulletin* 27, no. 1 (2001).

102. "Remarks by the First Lady at the White House Garden Harvest Party."

103. U.S. Department of Health, Education, and Welfare, *Obesity and Health: A Source Book of Current Information for Professional Health Personnel* (Washington, DC: U.S. Government Printing Office, 1966), 21.

104. *White House Conference on Food, Nutrition and Health: Final Report* (Washington, DC: U.S. Government Printing Office, 1969). Crandall et al., "An Attribution-Value Model of Prejudice."

105. Select Committee on Nutrition and Human Needs, United States Senate, *Dietary Goals for the United States*, 2nd ed. (Washington, DC: U.S. Government Printing Office, 1977), 7.

106. U.S. Department of Health and Human Services, *The Surgeon General's Call to Action to Prevent and Decrease Overweight and Obesity*, 12.

107. U.S. Department of Health and Human Services, *The Surgeon General's Call to Action to Prevent and Decrease Overweight and Obesity*, 13.

108. Jerome P. Kassirer and Marcia Angell, "Losing Weight: An Ill-Fated New Year's Resolution," *New England Journal of Medicine* 338, no. 1 (1998), 53.

109. Farrell, *Fat Shame*, 131; see chap. 3.

110. Robert Crawford, "The Boundaries of the Self and the Unhealthy Other: Reflections on Health, Culture and AIDS," *Social Science Medicine* 38, no. 10 (1994), 1359.

111. Crawford, "The Boundaries of the Self and the Unhealthy Other."

112. Brownell and Horgen, *Food Fight*, 42, 202–15.

113. Natalie Angier, "Who Is Fat?: It Depends on Culture," *New York Times*, November 7, 2000.

114. Weaver, Gaines, and Ebron, *Slim Down Sister*, 3. See also Zonda Hughes,

"Why So Many Black Women Are Overweight—and What They Can Do About It," *Ebony*, March 2000.

115. Saguy and Riley, "Weighing Both Sides," 887.

116. Saguy and Riley, "Weighing Both Sides," 870.

117. According to Kathleen LeBesco, "Anti-fat bias is more pronounced in individualist cultures that emphasize personal freedom and autonomous goal achievement. . . . The endorsement of a Protestant ethic ideology leads one to view stigmatized people as willful violates of traditional American values such as moral character, hard work, and self-discipline." LeBesco, *Revolting Bodies?*, 55.

118. Crandall et al., "An Attribution-Value Model of Prejudice." See also Diane M. Quinn and Jennifer Crocker, "When Ideology Hurts: Effects of Belief in the Protestant Ethic and Feeling Overweight on the Psychological Well-Being of Women," *Journal of Personality and Social Psychology* 77, no. 2 (1999).

119. Oliver, *Fat Politics*, 75.

120. Campos, *The Obesity Myth*, 4.

121. Weaver, Gaines, and Ebron, *Slim Down Sister*, 32.

122. Weaver, Gaines, and Ebron, *Slim Down Sister*, 32–33.

123. Robert Pool, *Fat: Fighting the Obesity Epidemic* (New York: Oxford University Press, 2001), 32.

124. Greg Critser, *Fat Land*, 129.

125. Understandings of minority obesity that focused on inherited differences drew on and reinforced the biological theories of race. Such views, while widely believed to have been eclipsed by social theories of racial difference starting in the early twentieth century, often lurked beneath social-constructionist veneers. For an interesting analysis of how biological notions of race pervade current thinking despite the supposed preeminence of cultural explanations, see Henry Yu, "How Tiger Woods Lost His Stripes: Post-Nationalist American Studies as a History of Race, Migration, and the Commodification of Culture," in *Post-Nationalist American Studies*, ed. John Carlos Rowe (Berkeley: University of California Press, 2000).

126. April Herndon observes, "It hardly seems a coincidence that at a time when medicalized or biologically based accounts of race and/or poverty have fallen out of vogue, arguments about the classed and raced nature of those hardest struck by the obesity epidemic have gained popularity." April Michelle Herndon, "Collateral Damage from Friendly Fire?: Race, Nation, Class and the 'War against Obesity,'" *Social Semiotics* 15, no. 2 (2005), 136.

127. Campos, *The Obesity Myth*, 82–83.

128. Critser, *Fat Land*, 131, 510–51.

129. Oliver, *Fat Politics*, 75.

130. See Farrell's *Fat Shame* for an excellent analysis of this dynamic both historically and in the present. LeBesco describes the presence of fat people "as the specter of downward mobility" and "disintegrating physical privilege." LeBesco, *Revolting Bodies?*, 56. Campos also notes that the affluent were "terrified" of obesity because "fat has the power, metaphorically speaking, to make us non-white and poor." Campos, *The Obesity Myth*, 69.

131. Tom Shadyac, dir., *The Nutty Professor* (Universal Pictures, 1996).

132. Pierre Bourdieu, *Distinction: A Social Critique of the Judgment of Taste* (Cambridge, MA: Harvard University Press, 1984).

133. Shadyac, *The Nutty Professor*.

134. Wann, "Fat Studies," xix–xxi.

135. Solovay, *Tipping the Scales of Justice*, 49.

136. Marilyn Wann, "BMI (Body Mass Index) = IMB (Imaginary Mental Barrier): Celebrating Weight Diversity via *Health at Every Size*," *Health at Every Size* (July–August 2004), 35.

SIX
Connecting the Dots: Dietary Reform Past, Present, and Future

1. Conversations with Amy Bentley and Aaron Bobrow-Strain helped shape my thinking about these connections. Carolyn de la Peña collaborated closely with me in writing my presentation, which was followed by her talk about what geography, anthropology, and sociology bring to the table. Thanks to Bruce German for the invitation.

2. Julie Guthman makes this point in regards to the alternative food movement, arguing for a "less messianic approach to food politics" and suggesting that activists should "do something different than 'invite others to the table,'" that has already been set. Julie Guthman, "If They Only Knew: Color Blindness and Universalism in California Alternative Food Institutions," *Professional Geographer* 60, no. 3 (2008), 388; Aaron Bobrow-Strain, *White Bread: A Social History of the Store-Bought Loaf* (Boston: Beacon, 2012), 12.

3. Danielle Boulé explores the social and cultural dimensions of healthy food access and barriers to access, especially those related to race and class, in her master's thesis "Beyond Black and White: Understanding the Sociocultural Dimensions of Healthy Food Access in South Sacramento," University of California, Davis, 2012.

4. Robert Crawford describes health as a fixation that "too often precludes discernment about the implications of its practice." He describes health as filling the void of a receding social sphere by providing meaning and purpose to life: "The social cynosure of health saturates the imagination with worries and tasks. Expansively, health becomes the 'what is to be done' of private life." Robert Crawford, "Health as Meaningful Social Practice," *Health* 10, no. 4 (2006), 404, 411.

5. Gyorgy Scrinis, "On the Ideology of Nutritionism," *Gastronomic* 8, no. 1 (2008); Michael Pollan, *In Defense of Food: An Eater's Manifesto* (New York: Penguin, 2008).

6. Marion Nestle, *Food Politics: How the Food Industry Influences Nutrition and Health* (Berkeley: University of California Press, 2002).

7. For more on the concept of "dietary literacy" see Biltekoff, "Critical Nutrition Studies" in *Handbook of Food History*, ed. Jeffrey Pilcher (New York: Oxford University Press), 2012.

8. Jay Mechling, "American Studies as a Social Movement," in *An American Mosaic: Rethinking American Culture Studies*, ed. M. W. Fishwick (New York: American Heritage, 1996), 25.

BIBLIOGRAPHY

Abel, Mary Hinman. "Proteid or Albuminous Food in Our Daily Fare." *The Rumford Kitchen Leaflets: Plain Words about Food*, ed. Ellen Richards. 68–72. Boston: Home Science Publishing, 1899.

——. "Public Kitchens in Relation to Workingmen and the Average Housewife." *The Rumford Kitchen Leaflets: Plain Words about Food*, ed. Ellen Richards. 155–60. Boston: Home Science Publishing, 1899.

——. "The Story of the New England Kitchen: Part 2, A Study in Social Economics." *The Rumford Kitchen Leaflets: Plain Words about Food*, ed. Ellen Richards. 131–54. Boston: Home Science Publishing, 1899.

"Alice's Restaurant." *Cooks Magazine*, 1983.

"Alice's Wonderland," *Newsweek* (August 27, 2001): 44–45.

"Alice Waters' Crusade for Better Food." *60 Minutes*. CBS, March 15, 2009.

Allen, Patricia. *Together at the Table: Sustainability and Sustenance in the American Agrifood System*. University Park: Pennsylvania State University Press/Rural Sociological Society, 2004.

Altheide, David L. "Consuming Terrorism." *Symbolic Interaction* 27, no. 3 (2004): 289–308.

——. *Terrorism and the Politics of Fear*. Lanham, MD: AltaMira Press, 2006.

Anderson, Karen. *Wartime Women: Sex Roles, Family Relations, and the Status of Women during World War II*. Westport, CT: Greenwood Press, 1981.

Angier, Natalie. "Who Is Fat?: It Depends on Culture." *New York Times*, November 7, 2000.

Atwater, W. O. "How Food Nourishes the Body: The Chemistry of Food and Nutrition II." *Century* (May–October 1887): 237–51.

——. "Pecuniary Economy of Food: The Chemistry of Foods and Nutrition V." *Century* (November 1887–April 1888): 437–46.

Atwater, W. O., and Charles D. Woods. *The Chemical Composition of American Food*

Materials. Washington, DC: U.S. Department of Agriculture, Office of Experiment Stations, 1899.

——. *Dietary Studies in New York City in 1895 and 1896, Bulletin No. 46*, ed. U.S. Department of Agriculture Office of Experiment Stations. Washington, DC: U.S.Government Printing Office, 1898.

Bahar, Zilah. "Personal Taste: Many Lessons Are Taught at the Edible Schoolyard." *San Francisco Examiner*, August 18, 1999.

Barret, Kate, and Brian Hartman. "Foodies Celebrate White House Veggie Garden." *ABC News*, March 20, 2009.

Barrows, Anna. "The Provision of Food for a Typical American Family." *American Kitchen* (October 1896): 27–28.

Belasco, Warren. *Appetite for Change: How the Counter Culture Took on the Food Industry, 1966–1988*. Ithaca, NY: Cornell University Press, 1989.

——. "Food, Morality, and Social Reform." *Morality and Health*, ed. Paul Rozin and Allen M. Brandt. 185–99. New York: Routledge, 1997.

Bentley, Amy. *Eating for Victory: Food Rationing and the Politics of Domesticity*. Urbana: University of Illinois Press, 1998.

Berry, Wendell. "Agricultural Solutions for Agricultural Problems." *Bringing It to the Table: On Farming and Food*. 19–30. Berkeley: Counterpoint, 2009.

——. "Land Use." *Last Whole Earth Catalog* (June 1971): 46.

——. "The Pleasure of Eating." *Bringing It to the Table: On Farming and Food*. 227–34. Berkeley: Counterpoint, 2009.

"Better Nutrition Sought by McNutt." *New York Times*, August 10, 1942.

Bevier, Isabel. "Mrs. Richards' Relation to the Home Economics Movement." *Journal of Home Economics* (June 1911): 214–16.

——. "The U.S. Government and the Housewife." *American Kitchen* (December 1898): 77–81.

Biltekoff, Charlotte. "Critical Nutrition Studies." *Handbook of Food History*, ed. Jeffrey Pilcher. New York: Oxford University Press, 2012.

——. "Functional Foods for Health: Negotiation and Implications," NABC Report 22, *Promoting Health by Linking Agriculture, Food, and Nutrition: Proceedings of the Twenty-second Annual Conference of the National Agricultural Biotechnology Council*, University of California, Davis, June 16–18, 2010, ed. Allan Eaglesham, Alan B. Bennet, and Ralph W. F. Hardy. 99–108. Ithaca, NY: National Agricultural Biotechnology Council, 2010.

——. "The Terror Within: Obesity in Post 9/11 U.S. Life." *American Studies* 48, no. 3 (fall 2008): 5–30.

Blumin, Stuart M. *The Emergence of the Middle Class: Social Experience in the American City, 1760–1900*. Cambridge: Cambridge University Press, 1989.

Bobrow-Strain, Aaron. *White Bread: A Social History of the Store-Bought Loaf*. Boston: Beacon, 2012.

Boulé, Danielle. "Beyond Black and White: Understanding the Sociocultural Dimensions of Healthy Food Access in South Sacramento." Master's thesis, University of California, Davis, 2012.

Bourdieu, Pierre. *Distinction: A Social Critique of the Judgment of Taste*. Cambridge, MA: Harvard University Press, 1984.

Braziel, Jana Evans, and Kathleen LeBesco, eds. *Bodies Out of Bounds: Fatness and Transgression*. Berkeley: University of California Press, 2001.

Brinkley, Alan. *The End of Reform*. New York: Alfred A. Knopf, 1995.

Brobeck, Florence. "Protective Foods for the Family." *New York Times*, March 8, 1936.

Brown, Ian. "Author Michael Pollan Explains the War on Food Movement." *Globe and Mail*, March 18, 2011. Available at http://www.theglobeandmail.com/life/author-michael-pollan-explains-the-war-on-food-movement/article573363.

Brownell, Kelly D., and Katherine Battle Horgen. *Food Fight: The Inside Story of the Food Industry, America's Obesity Crisis, and What We Can Do About It*. New York: McGraw-Hill, 2004.

Burbick, Joan. *Healing the Republic: The Language of Health and the Culture of Nationalism in Nineteenth-Century America*. Cambridge: Cambridge University Press, 1994.

Burres, Charles. "The Delicious Revolution Honored." *San Francisco Chronicle*, August 4, 1998.

Burros, Marian. "Obamas to Plant a Vegetable Garden at the White House." *New York Times*, March 20, 2009.

Bush, George W. "Remarks by the President on Fitness." Lakewest Family YMCA, Dallas, Texas, July 18, 2003. Available at http://georgewbush-whitehouse.archives.gov/news/releases/2003/07/20030718–6.html.

Campos, Paul. *The Obesity Myth: Why America's Obsession with Weight Is Hazardous to Your Health*. New York: Gotham Books, 2004.

Carmona, Richard. "Remarks at the American Enterprise Institute Obesity Conference." U.S. Department of Health and Human Services, Washington, DC, June 10, 2003. Available at http://www.surgeongeneral.gov/news/speeches/obesity061003.html.

——. "Remarks to the California Childhood Obesity Conference." U.S. Department of Health and Human Services, January 6, 2003. Available at http://www.surgeongeneral.gov/news/speeches/califobesity.html.

Chittenden, R. H. "The Digestibility of Proteid Foods." *The Rumford Kitchen Leaflets: Plain Words about Food*, ed. Ellen H. Richards. 63–67. Boston: Home Science Publishing, 1899.

Clemen, Jane, Diana Kirkwood, Bobbi Schell, and Daniel Myerson. *The Town that Lost a Ton: How One Town Used the Buddy System to Lose 3,998 Pounds . . . and How You Can Too!* Naperville, IL: Sourcebooks, 2002.

Committee on Food Habits. "Manual for the Study of Food Habits." *Report of the Committee on Food Habits*. Washington, DC: National Research Council, 1945.

——. "The Problem of Changing Food Habits: Report of the Committee on Food Habits 1941–1943." *Bulletin of the National Research Council Number 108*. Washington, DC: National Research Council, 1943.

Committee on Nutrition in Industry, National Research Council. *The Food and Nu-*

trition of Industrial Workers in Wartime. Washington, DC: National Research Council, 1942.

Committee on Nutrition of Industrial Workers, Food and Nutrition Board. *The Nutrition of Industrial Workers*. Second report of the Committee on Nutrition of Industrial Workers. Washington, DC: National Research Council, 1945.

Consumer Counsel Division of the United States Department of Agriculture. "Food and National Defense Issue." *Consumer's Guide* 6, no. 20 (1943).

——. "Mrs. America Volunteers." Special issue, *Consumer's Guide* 7, no. 20 (October 15, 1941).

Cooke, Kathy J. "The Limits of Heredity: Nature and Nurture in American Eugenics before 1915." *Journal of the History of Biology* 31 (1998): 263–78.

Coveney, John. *Food, Morals, and Meaning: The Pleasure and Anxiety of Eating*. New York: Routledge, 2000.

——. *Food, Morals, and Meaning: The Pleasure and Anxiety of Eating*. 2nd ed. New York: Routledge, 2006.

Craig, Hazel T. *The History of Home Economics*. New York: Practical Home Economics, 1946.

Crandall, Christian S., S. D'Anello, N. Sakalli, E. Lazarus, G. W. Nejtardt, N. T. Feather. "An Attribution-Value Model of Prejudice: Anti-Fat Attitudes in Six Nations." *Personality and Social Psychology Bulletin* 27, no. 1 (2001): 30–37.

Crane, Elizabeth. "The Incredible, Edible Schoolyard: School Garden Projects Are Reaping the Benefits of Teaching Community Values and Hands-On Learning." *District Administration* July 2003. Available at http://www.districtadministration.com/article/incredible-edible-schoolyard.

Crawford, Robert. "The Boundaries of the Self and the Unhealthy Other: Reflections on Health, Culture and AIDS." *Social Science Medicine* 38, no. 10 (1994): 1347–65.

——. "A Cultural Account of 'Health': Control, Release, and the Social Body." *Issues on the Political Economy of Health Care*, ed. John B. McKinley. 60–103. New York: Tavistock, 1984.

——. "Health as Meaningful Social Practice." *Health* 10, no. 4 (2006): 401–20.

——. "Healthism and the Medicalization of Everyday Life." *International Journal of Health Services* 10, no. 3 (1980): 365–88.

Critser, Greg. *Fat Land: How Americans Became the Fattest People in the World*. Boston: Houghton Mifflin, 2003.

Crotty, Patricia. *Good Nutrition?: Fact and Fashion in Dietary Advice*. St. Leonards, Australia: Allen and Unwin, 1995.

Cullather, Nick. "The Foreign Policy of the Calorie." *American Historical Review* 112, no. 2 (2007): 337–64.

Cummings, Richard Osborn. *The American and His Food: A History of Food Habits in the United States*. Chicago: University of Chicago Press, 1940.

Davis, Ethel. "Dishonesty in Caste and in House-Furnishing." *New England Kitchen* (September 1894): 269–72.

——. "Dishonesty and Caste in Housekeeping and Home-Making." *New England Kitchen* (January 1895): 169–74.

Democracy Means All of Us. Washington, DC: Federal Security Agency, Office of Defense Health and Welfare Services, 1943.

Dietz, William H., Barbara Browman, James S. Marks, and Jeffrey P. Koplan. "The Spread of the Obesity Epidemic in the United States." *Journal of the American Medical Association* 282, no. 16 (October 1999): 1519–22.

Division of Campaigns, Office of War Information, in Cooperation with Nutrition Division of Health and Welfare Services. *Better Health: A Speedier Victory through Proper Nutrition*. Book 6 of the U.S. Government Campaign to Promote the Production, Sharing and Proper Use of Food. Washington, DC: U.S. Government Printing Office, 1943.

Duis, Perry R. "No Time for Privacy: World War II and Chicago's Families." *The War in American Culture: Society and Consciousness during World War II*, ed. Lewis A. Erenberg and Susan E. Hirsch. 17–45. Chicago: University of Chicago Press, 1996.

"Eating Less Urged for Those over 25: Obesity a National Malady." *New York Times*, April 17, 1952.

Epstein, Barbara Leslie. *The Politics of Domesticity: Women, Evangelism, and Temperance in Nineteenth-Century America*. Middletown, CT: Wesleyan University Press, 1981.

Erenberg, Lewis A., and Susan E. Hirsch, eds. *The War in American Culture: Society and Consciousness during World War II*. Chicago: University of Chicago Press, 1996.

Farrell, Amy Erdman. *Fat Shame: Stigma and the Fat Body in American Culture*. New York: New York University Press, 2011.

"First Lady Appeals for Unified People." *New York Times*, November 18, 1941.

Flegal, Katherine M., Barry I. Graubard, David F. Williamson, and Mitchell H. Gail. "Excess Deaths Associated with Underweight, Overweight, and Obesity." *Journal of the American Medical Association* 293, no. 15 (April 20, 2005): 1861–67.

Flegal, Katherine M., and R. J. Kuczymarski. "Criteria for Definition of Overweight in Transition: Background and Recommendations for the United States." *American Journal of Clinical Nutrition* 72 (2000): 1974–81.

Flegal, Katherine M., David Williamson, Elsie Pamuk, and Harry M. Rosenberg. "Estimating Deaths Attributable to Obesity in the United States." *American Journal of Public Health* 94, no. 9 (September 2004): 1486–89.

Food and Nutrition Board Committee on Diagnosis and Pathology of Nutritional Deficiencies. "Inadequate Diets and Nutritional Deficiencies in the United States: Their Prevalence and Significance." *Bulletin of the National Research Council Number 109*. Washington, DC: National Research Council, 1943.

"Foods Prepared and Sold at the Rumford Kitchen, with Their Food Values." *The Rumford Kitchen Leaflets: Plain Words about Food*, ed. Ellen Richards. 15. Boston: Home Science Publishing, 1899.

Fumento, Michael. "Obesity Is Contagious." *American Spectator* (August 1, 2007). Available at http://spectator.org/archives/2007/08/01/obesity-is-contagious.

Gawande, Atul. "The Man Who Couldn't Stop Eating." *New Yorker* (July 9, 2001, 66–75.

General Mills. *General Mills Nutrition Study Kit*. Minneapolis: General Mills, 1941.
Ginzberg, Lori D. *Women and the Work of Benevolence: Morality, Politics and Class in the Nineteenth-Century United States*. New Haven, CT: Yale University Press, 1990.
Gleason, Philip. "Pluralism, Democracy and Catholicism in the Era of World War II." *Review of Politcs* 49, no. 2 (spring 1987): 208–30.
Goodhart, Robert. "Wartime Feeding of Industrial Workers." *Nutrition and the Food Supply: The War and After*, ed. John D. Black. 225:116–21. *Annals of the American Academy of Political and Social Science*. Philadelphia: American Academy of Political and Social Science, 1943.
Goodrich, Henrietta. "Suggestions for a Professional School of Home and Social Economics." *Proceedings of the First, Second, and Third Conferences*, by Lake Placid Conference on Home Economics, 26–44. Lake Placid, NY: American Home Economics Association, 1899–1901.
Graebner, William. *The Engineering of Consent: Democracy and Authority in Twentieth-Century America*. Madison: University of Wisconsin Press, 1987.
"Guide to the Rumford Kitchen." *The Rumford Kitchen Leaflets: Plain Words about Food*, ed. Ellen Richards. 11–15. Boston: Home Science Publishing, 1899.
Gussow, Joan Dye. *The Feeding Web: Issues in Nutritional Ecology*. Palo Alto, CA: Bull Publishing, 1978.
——. "Growth, Truth, and Responsibility: Food Is the Bottom Line." *Ellen Swallow Richards Lecture Series*. 1–15. Greensboro: Institute of Nutrition, University of North Carolina, 1981.
——. "PCBs for Breakfast and Other Problems of a Food System Gone Awry." *Food Monitor* (May–June 1982): 16–19, 28.
——. *This Organic Life: Confessions of a Surburban Homesteader*. White River Junction, VT: Chelsea Green Publishing, 2001.
Guthman, Julie. *Agrarian Dreams: The Paradox of Organic Farming in California*. Berkeley: University of California Press, 2004.
——. "Can't Stomach It: How Michael Pollan et al. Made Me Want to Eat Cheetos." *Gastronomica* (summer 2007): 75–79.
——. "Fast Food/Organic Food: Reflexive Tastes and the Making of 'Yuppie Chow.'" *Social and Cultural Geography* 4, no. 1 (2003): 46–58.
——. "If They Only Knew: Color Blindness and Universalism in California Alternative Food Institutions." *Professional Geographer* 60, no. 3 (2008): 387–97.
——. "Neoliberalism and the Constitution of Contemporary Bodies." *The Fat Studies Reader*, ed. Sondra Solovay and Esther Rothblum. 187–96. New York: New York University Press, 2009.
——. "Neoliberalism and the Making of Food Politics in California." *Geoforum* 39, no. 3 (2008): 1171–83.
——. *Weighing In: Obesity, Food Justice, and the Limits of Capitalism*. Berkeley: University of California Press, 2011.
Guthman, Julie, and Patricia Allen. "From 'Old School' to 'Farm-to-School': Neoliberalism from the Ground Up." *Agriculture and Human Values* 23 (2006): 401–15.

Harvey, David. *A Brief History of Neoliberalism*. New York: Oxford University Press, 2005.

Hasler, Clare. "The Changing Face of Functional Foods." *Journal of the American College of Nutrition* 19, no. 5 (2000): 499s–506s.

Hays, Samuel P. *The Response to Industrialism 1885–1914*. 2nd ed. Chicago: University of Chicago Press, 1995.

Healy, Melissa. "War on Fat Gets Serious." *Los Angeles Times*, January 3, 2004.

Hegsted, David Mark. "Recollections of a Pioneer in Nutrition: Fifty Years in Nutrition." *Journal of the College of Nutrition* 9, no. 4 (1990): 280–87.

Hellmich, Nanci. "Fat Is in Your BMI, but Also in the Eye of the Beholder." *USA Today*, June 10, 1998.

Herndon, April Michelle. "Collateral Damage from Friendly Fire?: Race, Nation, Class and the 'War against Obesity.'" *Social Semiotics* 15, no. 2 (August 2005): 128–41.

Hoffman, Lisa. "Half of U.S. Military Population Overweight, Study Says: A Few Extra Pounds Likely to Affect Combat Readiness of a Few Good Men." *Washington Times*, January 1, 2002.

Horowitz, Howard. "Always With Us." *American Literary History* 10, no. 2 (summer 1998): 317–34.

Hughes, Zonda. "Why So Many Black Women Are Overweight—and What They Can Do About It." *Ebony* (March 2000): 92–96.

Hunt, Caroline L. *The Life of Ellen Richards*. Boston: Whitcomb and Barrows, 1912.

International Labour Office. *Nutrition in Industry*. Montreal: International Labour Office, 1946.

"Interview with Surgeon General Richard Carmona." *Morning Edition*, National Public Radio, November 27, 2003.

Ives, Susan. "Feeding Hearts and Minds: Interview: Alice Waters." *Land and People* (fall 1999). Available at http://www.tpl.org/publications/land-and-people-magazine/archive/landpeople-fall-1999/feeding-hearts-and-minds.html.

Jackson, Derrick Z. "All Quiet on the Fat Front." *Boston Globe*, October 11, 2002.

Johaness, Laura, and Steve Stecklow. "Dire Warnings about Obesity Rely on Slippery Statistics." *Wall Street Journal*, February 9, 1998.

Jones, Irma. "Ethics of the Kitchen." *New England Kitchen* (December 1894): 109–12.

Julier, Alice. "How Not to Define Your Social Movement: Notes on Feminism, Intersectionality, and Food." Paper presented at the "Food Networks: Gender and Foodways" conference. University of Notre Dame Gender Studies Program, Notre Dame, Indiana, January 26–28, 2012.

Jung, Ted. *For Work, for Play, 3 'Squares' a Day: Eat the Basic 7 Way*. Washington, DC: U.S. Government Printing Office, 1944.

Kamminga, Harmke. "Nutrition for the People, or the Fate of Jacob Moleschott's Contest for a Humanist Science." *The Science and Culture of Nutrition, 1840–1940*, ed. Harmke Kamminga and Andrew Cunningham. 15–48. Amsterdam: Rodopi, 1995.

Kamminga, Harmke, and Andrew Cunningham. "Introduction: The Science and Culture of Nutrition, 1840–1940." *The Science and Culture of Nutrition, 1840–1940*,

ed. Harmke Kamminga and Andrew Cunningham. 1–14. Amsterdam: Rodopi, 1995.
Kassirer, Jerome P., and Marcia Angell. "Losing Weight: An Ill-Fated New Year's Resolution." *New England Journal of Medicine* 338, no. 1 (January 1, 1998): 52–54.
Kasson, John F. "Rituals of Dining: Table Manners in Victorian America." *Dining in America, 1850–1900*, ed. Kathryn Grover. 114–42. Rochester, NY: Margaret Woodbury Strong Museum, 1987.
Kelley, Ken. "Alice Waters." *Mother Jones*, January–February 1995. Available at http://www.motherjones.com/politics/1995/01/alice-waters.
Kingsolver, Barbara, Steven L. Hopp, and Camille Kingsolver. *Animal, Vegetable, Miracle: A Year of Food Life*. New York: HarperCollins, 2007.
Kolata, Gina. "The Fat Epidemic: He Says It's an Illusion." *New York Times*, June 8, 2004.
——. "Longing to Lose, at a Cost." *New York Times*, January 4, 2005.
Koop, C. Everett. "Dr. C. Everett Koop Launches a New 'Crusade' to Combat Obesity in America." Shape Up America!, December 6, 1994. Available at http://www.shapeup.org/about/arch_pr/120694.php.
Kwan, Samantha. "Individual Versus Corporate Responsibility." *Food, Culture and Society* 12, no. 4 (December 2009): 477–95.
Lake Placid Conference on Home Economics. *Proceedings of the First, Second and Third Conferences*." Lake Placid, NY: American Home Economics Association, 1901.
——. *Proceedings of the Fourth Conference*. Lake Placid, NY: American Home Economics Association, 1902.
——. *Proceedings of the Sixth Conference*. Lake Placid, NY: American Home Economics Association, 1904.
Lambert, Craig. "The Way We Eat Now: Ancient Bodies Collide with Modern Technology to Produce a Flabby, Disease-Ridden Populace." *Harvard Magazine* (May–June 2004): 48–58, 98–99.
Lappé, Frances Moore. *Diet for a Small Planet*. New York: Ballantine, 1971.
——. "Food, Farming and Democracy." *Our Sustainable Table*, ed. Robert Clark, 143–60. San Francisco: North Point Press, 1990.
Lawrence, Mark, and Mike Rayner. "Functional Foods and Health Claims: A Public Health Policy Perspective." *Public Health Nutrition* 1, no. 2 (1998): 75–82.
LeBesco, Kathleen. "Neoliberalism, Public Health, and the Moral Perils of Fatness." *Critical Public Health* (2010): 1–12.
——. *Revolting Bodies?: The Struggle to Redefine Fat Identity*. Amherst: University of Massachusetts Press, 2004.
Lee, Taeku, and Eric J. Oliver. "Public Opinion and the Politics of America's Obesity Epidemic." Social Science Research Network, May 2002. Available at http://papers.ssrn.com/s013/papers.cfm?abstract_id=313824.
Levenstein, Harvey. *Paradox of Plenty: A Social History of Eating in Modern America*. New York: Oxford University Press, 1993.

——. *Revolution at the Table: The Transformation of the American Diet*. New York: Oxford University Press, 1988.

Lewin, Kurt. "Forces behind Food Habits and Methods of Change," in Committee on Food Habits, *The Problem of Changing Food Habits: Report of the Committee on Food Habits 1941–1943, Bulletin of the National Research Council No. 108* (October 1943): 35–65.

Lupton, Deborah. *Food, the Body and the Self*. London: Sage, 1996.

Lupton, Deborah, and Alan Petersen. *The New Public Health: Health and Self in the Age of Risk*. London: Sage, 1996.

Lyons, Pat. "Prescription for Harm: Diet Industry Influence, Public Health, and the 'Obesity Epidemic.'" *The Fat Studies Reader*, ed. Sondra Solovay and Esther Rothblum. 75–87. New York: New York University Press, 2009.

McNamee, Thomas. *Alice Waters and Chez Panisse*. New York: Penguin, 2007.

"McNutt Takes Up New Defense Task." *New York Times*, December 4, 1940.

Mechling, Jay. "American Studies as a Social Movement." *An American Mosaic: Rethinking American Culture Studies*, ed. M. W. Fishwick. 15–26. New York: American Heritage, 1996.

Mudry, Jessica. *Measured Meals: Nutrition in America*. Albany: State University of New York Press, 2009.

Mulligan, Megan. "Michelle Obama to Create an Organic 'Victory' Garden at the White House." *Guardian*, March 20, 2009. Available at http://www.guardiannews.com.

National Body Challenge. Discovery Health Channel, 2004.

Nestle, Marion. *Food Politics: How the Food Industry Influences Nutrition and Health*. Berkeley: University of California Press, 2002.

New York State College of Home Economics, Department of Food and Nutrition. "Records #23/14/2485." Division of Rare and Manuscript Collections, Cornell University.

Nissenbaum, Stephen. *Sex, Diet, and Debility in Jacksonian America: Sylvester Graham and Health Reform*. Westport, CT: Greenwood Press, 1980.

"Nurturing Connections with Farmers: An Interview with Alice Waters." *In Season: A Report on Locally Grown Produce* (1997). Available at http://marketreport.com/waters.htm.

O'Neill, Molly. "Keeper of the Flame." *New York Times Magazine* (December 12, 1992): 29–30.

Oliver, Eric J. *Fat Politics: The Real Story behind America's Obesity Epidemic*. New York: Oxford University Press, 2006.

"Overeating Called 'Compulsive': Diet Held Only Way to Reduce." *New York Times*, October 21, 1950.

"Overeating Laid to U.S." *New York Times*, April 4, 1950.

Parloa, Maria. "The New England Kitchen." *Century* (December 1891): 315–17.

Peck, J., and A. Tickell. "Neoliberalizing Space." *Antipode* 43, no. 3 (2002): 380–404.

Pivar, David. *Purity Crusade: Sexual Morality and Social Control, 1868–1900*. Westport, CT: Greenwood Press, 1973.

Pollan, Michael. *Food Rules: An Eater's Manifesto*. New York: Penguin, 2009.
——. *In Defense of Food: An Eater's Manifesto*. New York: Penguin, 2008.
——. *The Omnivore's Dilemma: A Natural History of Four Meals*. New York: Penguin, 2006.
——. "The Way We Live Now: The (Agri)Cultural Contradictions of Obesity." *New York Times Magazine* (October 12, 2003). Available at http://www.nytimes.com/2003/10/12/magazine/12WWLN.html?pagewanted=all.
——. "Why Eating Well Is 'Elitist,'" *New York Times* "On the Table Blog," May 11, 2006. http://michaelpollan.com/articles-archive/why-eating-well-is-elitist/.
Pollan, Michael, and Maira Kalman. *Food Rules: An Eater's Manual*. New York: Penguin, 2011.
Pool, Robert. *Fat: Fighting the Obesity Epidemic*. New York: Oxford University Press, 2001.
Proceedings of the National Nutrition Conference for Defense. Washington, DC: Federal Security Agency, Office of the Director of Defense, Health and Welfare Services, 1941.
Pudup, Mary Beth. "It Takes a Garden: Cultivating Citizen-Subjects in Organized Garden Projects." *Geoforum* 39, no. 3 (2008): 1228–40.
Quinn, Diane M., and Jennifer Crocker. "When Ideology Hurts: Effects of Belief in the Protestant Ethic and Feeling Overweight on the Psychological Well-Being of Women." *Journal of Personality and Social Psychology* 77, no. 2 (1999): 410–14.
Radhakrishnan, Bharathi. "Can Air Conditioning Make You Fat?," June 27, 2006. Available at http://abcnews.go.com/Health/Diet/story?id=2120381&page=1.
Rauber, Paul. "Conservation à la Carte." *Sierra* 79, no. 6 (November–December 1994): 42–52.
"Remarks by the First Lady at the White House Garden Harvest Party." White House Office of the First Lady, June 16, 2009. Available at http://www.whitehouse.gov/the-press-office/remarks-first-lady-white-house-garden-harvest-party.
Report on Nutrition Activities 1941–1942. Ithaca: New York State College of Home Economics, 1942.
Reuben, Julie A. "Beyond Politics: Community Civics and the Redefinition of Citizenship in the Progressive Era." *History of Education Quarterly* 37, no. 4 (winter 1997): 399–420.
Reuters. "U.S. Male Soldiers Are Getting Fatter." *San Diego Union-Tribune*, November 10, 2001.
Rice, Marjorie. "Chefs: War and Peas." *San Francisco Examiner*, December 30, 1992.
Richards, Ellen. *The Art of Right Living*. Boston: Whitcomb and Barrows, 1904.
——. *The Cost of Food: A Study of Dietaries*. New York: J. Wiley and Sons, 1901.
——. "Euthenics in Higher Education: Better Living Conditions." *Proceedings of the Eighth Conference*, by Lake Placid Conference on Home Economics. 33–35. Lake Placid, NY: American Home Economics Association, 1906.
——. *Euthenics: The Science of a Controllable Environment*. Boston: Whitcomb and Barrows, 1910.

———. "The Foods of Institutions." *The Rumford Kitchen Leaflets: Plain Words about Food*, ed. Ellen Richards. 166–73. Boston: Home Science Publishing, 1899.
———. "Good Food for Little Money." *The Rumford Kitchen Leaflets: Plain Words about Food*, ed. Ellen Richards. 123–31. Boston: Home Science Publishing, 1899.
———. "Luncheons for School." *New England Kitchen* (May 1895): 51–54.
———. "Nomenclature." *Proceedings of the Sixth Conference*, by Lake Placid Conference on Home Economics, 63–64. Lake Placid, NY: American Home Economics Association, 1904.
———, ed. *The Rumford Kitchen Leaflets: Plain Words about Food*. Boston: Home Science Publishing, 1899.
———. "Social Significance of the Home Economics Movement." *Journal of Home Economics* 3, no. 2 (1911): 117–25.
Roberts, Lydia J. "Beginning of the Recommended Dietary Allowances." *Journal of the American Dietetic Association* 34, no. 9 (1958): 33–38.
Rosenberg, Charles E. *No Other Gods: On Science and American Social Thought*. Baltimore: Johns Hopkins University Press, 1961.
Rosenblatt, Robert A. "Surgeon General Takes Stern Stance on Obesity." *Los Angeles Times*, December 14, 2001.
Rusk, Howard A. "Overweight Persons Termed Top Health Problem in U.S." *New York Times*, April 17, 1952.
Saguy, Abigail C., and Kevin W. Riley. "Weighing Both Sides: Morality, Mortality, and Framing Contests over Obesity." *Journal of Health Politics, Policy and Law* 30, no. 5 (2005): 869–921.
Samuel, Lawrence R. *Pledging Allegiance: American Identity and the Bond Drive of World War II*. Washington, DC: Smithsonian Institution Press, 1997.
Schlosser, Eric. *Fast Food Nation: The Dark Side of the All-American Meal*. Boston: Houghton Mifflin, 2001.
Scrinis, Gyorgy. *Nutritionism: The Science and Politics of Dietary Advice*. New York: Columbia University Press, 2013.
———. "On the Ideology of Nutritionism." *Gastronomic* 8, no. 1 (2008): 39–48.
———. "Sorry, Marge." *Meanjin* 61, no. 4 (2002): 108–16.
Sedgwick, W. T. "On External Digestion Commonly Called Alimentation." *The Rumford Kitchen Leaflets: Plain Words about Food*, ed. Ellen Richards, 45–50. Boston: Home Science Publishing, 1899.
Seid, Roberta Pollack. *Never Too Thin: Why Women Are at War with Their Bodies*. New York: Prentice Hall, 1989.
Select Committee on Nutrition and Human Needs, U.S. Senate. *Dietary Goals for the United States*. 2nd ed. Washington, DC: U.S. Government Printing Office, 1977.
Severson, Kim. "Obesity 'a Threat' to U.S. Security: Surgeon General Urges Cultural Shift." *San Francisco Chronicle*, January 7, 2003.
Shadyac, Tom, dir. *The Nutty Professor*. Universal Pictures, 1996.
Shapiro, Laura. *Perfection Salad: Women and Cooking at the Turn of the Century*. New York: Henry Holt, 1986.
———. "The War on Alice Waters." *Gourmet*, May 6, 2009.

Singer, Michael. "Fat of the Land." *New York Times Magazine* (April 3, 2001): 22.
Slocum, Rachel. "Whiteness, Space and Alternative Food Practice." *Geoform* 38 (2007): 520–33.
Solovay, Sondra. *Tipping the Scales of Justice: Fighting Weight-Based Discrimination*. Amherst, NY: Prometheus Books, 2000.
Solovay, Sondra, and Esther Rothblum, eds. *The Fat Studies Reader*. New York: New York University Press, 2009.
Stage, Sarah. "Ellen Richards and the Social Significance of the Home Economics Movement." *Rethinking Home Economics: Women and the History of a Profession*, ed. Sarah Stage and Virginia B. Vincenti. 17–33. Ithaca, NY: Cornell University Press, 1997.
Stanley, Louise. "Science of Nutrition at the Home Base." *The Family in a World at War*, ed. Sidonie Matznder Gruenberg. 46–55. New York: Harper Brothers, 1942.
Starrett, Helen Ekin. "The Home and the Labor Problem." *New England Kitchen* (February 1895): 239–41.
Stearns, Peter. *Fat History: Bodies and Beauty in the Modern West*. New York: New York University Press, 1997.
Stiebeling, Hazel. "Family Food Consumption and Dietary Levels: Five Regions." *U.S. Department of Agriculture Misc. Pub. no. 405*. Washington, DC: U.S. Government Printing Office, 1941.
"Superflour." *New York Times*, January 12, 1941.
Superville, Darlene. "Ground Is Broken for White House 'Kitchen Garden.'" *SFGate*, March 20, 2009. Available at http://www.sfgate.com.
"Surgeon General to Cops: Put Down the Donuts." CNN.com, March 2, 2003. Available at http://www.cnn.com/2003/health/02/28/obesity.police.
Sweeny, Mary. "Changing Food Habits." *Journal of Home Economics* 43, no. 7 (1942): 457–62.
Thurs, Daniel Patrick. *Science Talk: Changing Notions of Science in American Culture*. New Brunswick, NJ: Rutgers University Press, 2008.
Tomes, Nancy. "Moralizing the Microbe: The Germ Theory and the Moral Construction of Behavior in the Late-Nineteenth-Century Antituberculosis Movement." *Morality and Health*, ed. Allen M. Brandt and Paul Rozin. 271–94. New York: Routledge, 1997.
Ulmer, Marion Jordan. "Feeding Four on a Dollar a Day." Denver: Marion Jordan Ulmer, 1942.
United States Department of Agriculture, Bureau of Agricultural Economics. *Nutrition and the War: Opinions about Food, and Their Significance for Better Nutrition*. Washington, DC: U.S. Government Printing Office, 1943.
United States Department of Agriculture, War Food Administration, Nutrition and Food Conservation Branch. *Manual of Industrial Nutrition*. Washington, DC: U.S. Government Printing Office, 1943.
United States Department of Health and Human Services. *The Surgeon General's Call to Action to Prevent and Decrease Overweight and Obesity*. Rockland, MD: U.S. De-

partment of Health and Human Services, Public Health Service, Office of the Surgeon General, 2001.

United States Department of Health, Education, and Welfare. *Obesity and Health: A Source Book of Current Information for Professional Health Personnel*. Washington, DC: U.S. Government Printing Office, 1966.

Veit, Helen Zoe. "'We Were a Soft People': Asceticism, Self-Discipline and American Food Conservation in the First World War." *Food, Culture and Society* 10, no. 2 (summer 2007): 167–90.

Wade, Mary L. "Healthful and Economical Foods." *New England Kitchen* (April 1896): 33–35.

Wann, Marilyn. "BMI (Body Mass Index) = IMB (Imaginary Mental Barrier): Celebrating Weight Diversity via *Health at Every Size*." *Health at Every Size* (July–August 2004): 35–36.

——. "Fat Studies: An Invitation to Revolution." *The Fat Studies Reader*, ed. Sondra Solovay and Esther Rothblum, xi–xxvi. New York: New York University Press, 2009.

War Information Program. *Food Fights for Freedom*. Report prepared by the Office of Program Coordination, Office of War Information, and War Food Administration, in cooperation with Office of Price Administration, 1943.

Waters, Alice. "The Delicious Revolution." Paper presented at the Environmental Grantmakers Association 1999 Retreat, Pacific Grove, California, October 25, 1999.

——. "The Ethics of Eating." Paper presented at the Mills College Commencement, Oakland, California, May 22, 1994.

——. "The Ethics of Eating: Part Two." Paper presented at the Sixteenth Annual Ecological Farming Conference, Asilomar, California, January 25, 1996.

——. "The Farm-Restaurant Connection." *Our Sustainable Table*, ed. Robert Clark, 113–24. San Francisco: North Point Press, 1990.

——. "Fast Food Values." Keynote address at REAP conference, Madison, Wisconsin, September 2002.

——. "A Letter to Clinton and Gore." December 9, 1995. *EarthLight*. Available at http://www.earthlight.org/alicewaters23.html.

——. "Making Food the Educational Priority." Paper presented at the American Institute of Food and Wine conference "Children's Education: Feeding Our Future," Monterrey, California, March 10–13, 1994.

——. "Slow Food, Slow Schools: Teaching Sustainability through the Education of the Senses." Paper presented at the program in agrarian studies at Yale University, New Haven, Connecticut, 2003.

——. "Slow Food, Slow Schools: Transforming Education through a School Lunch Curriculum." October 2003. www.edibleschoolyard.org/Alice_message.html.

——. "Speech to the Baker's Guild." Paper presented at the REAP Conference, Madison, Wisconsin, September 1998.

Waters, Alice, Linda P. Guenzel, and Carolyn Dille. *The Chez Panisse Menu Cookbook*. New York: Random House, 1982.

Waters, Alice, Alan Tangren, and Fritz Streiff. *Chez Panisse Fruit*. New York: HarperCollins, 2002.

Weaver, Roniece, Fabiola D. Gaines, and Angela Ebron. *Slim Down Sister: The African American Woman's Guide to Healthy, Permanent Weight Loss*. New York: Dutton, 2000.

Wee, Christina C., Mary B. Hamel, Roger B. Davis, and Russell S. Phillips. "Assessing the Value of Weight Loss among Primary Care Patients." *Journal of General Internal Medicine* 19 (2004): 1206–11.

Weibe, Robert H. *The Search for Order, 1877–1920*. New York: Hill and Wang, 1967.

Weingarten, Tara. "Alice's Wonderland." *Newsweek* (August 27, 2001): 44–45.

White House Conference on Food, Nutrition and Health: Final Report. Washington, DC: U.S. Government Printing Office, 1969.

Whorton, James C. *Crusaders for Fitness: The History of American Health Reformers*. Princeton, NJ: Princeton University Press, 1982.

Wile, Ira S. "School Lunches." *Journal of Home Economics* (April 1910): 160–69.

Wilkins, Walter, and French Boyd. *Nutrition for You!* (1943). Available at http://hdl.handle.net/2027/coo.31924003554.

Winkler, Allan M. *Home Front U.S.A.: America during World War Two*. Arlington Heights, IL: Harlan Davidson, 1986.

Witt, Linda. "Stirring Up a Cooking Revolution." *Chicago Tribune Sunday Magazine* (May 11, 1986).

Yu, Henry. "How Tiger Woods Lost His Stripes: Post-Nationalist American Studies as a History of Race, Migration, and the Commodification of Culture." *Post-Nationalist American Studies*, ed. John Carlos Rowe. 223–46. Berkeley: University of California Press, 2000.

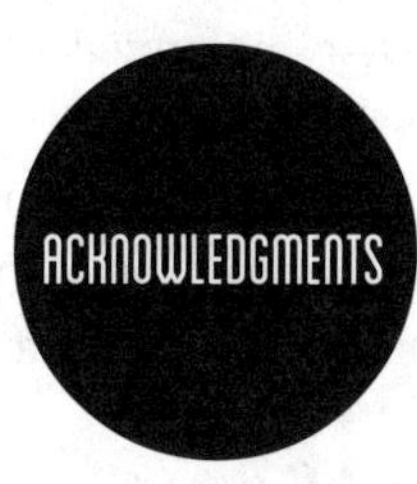

ACKNOWLEDGMENTS

This book has been part of my life for so long, it would be impossible to thank every person who in some way made it possible. My long trail of debt and gratitude starts with the people who nurtured my early interest in food and set me on my path: my friends at Green's Restaurant, especially Jay Kenyon and Annie Somerville, who took a chance on me and taught me how to taste and talk about food; Jonathan D. Katz, who took me into the hallway during a San Francisco City College class and told me to go back to college; and my mentors at the University of California (UC), Berkeley, Kathleen Moran and Margaretta Lovell, who took my interest in food seriously, oversaw the undergraduate thesis that later became the dissertation that eventually became this book, and sent me on my way to graduate school.

At Brown University, I had the great fortune to work with advisors who, though they did not study food themselves, never doubted the seriousness of my scholarship and who helped me gather the tools I needed to answer the questions I cared about. Thank you, Nancy Armstrong, Carolyn Dean, and especially Mari Jo Buhle, whose experience as a trailblazer in the field of women's history gave me confidence when I needed it most.

I attended my first meeting of the Association for the Study of Food and Society in 1996, just before I started graduate school. The fact that I finished this project and with my sanity, sense of humor, and intellect relatively intact is a testament to the countless friends and colleagues—far too many to thank each by name—that I have found there over the years.

Alice Julier has sustained me with her intelligence, spirit, wit and drive since I was fortunate enough to meet her at that very first meeting. Warren Belasco has been a steadfast mentor and friend, generously guiding me through the endless process of professionalization. As a reviewer for Duke, he provided manuscript feedback that was full of his characteristic warmth, sharpness, and wisdom. I also want to specially thank Amy Bentley, Netta Davis, Lisa Heldke, Elaine Power, Christie Shields-Argelès, Psyche Williams-Forson, and Abby Wilkerson for their guidance, humor, and intellectual exchange over the years.

UC Davis has provided many opportunities for professional growth for which I am very grateful. I want to thank all of my colleagues in food science and technology, especially those whose bold visions for interdisciplinary exchange have presented me with the challenges I needed to grow into the kind of scholar I most want to be: Charlie Bamforth, Christine Bruhn, Bruce German, Jean-Xavier Guinard, Clare Hasler, John Krochta, Kathryn McCarthy, Mike McCarthy, and Carl Winter. I am extremely lucky to have colleagues in American studies who are exceptionally likeable and cooperative, and I want to extend special thanks to my chairs, Eric Smoodin and Julie Sze, for their guidance. The Davis Humanities Institute has provided opportunities to learn from people from across the social sciences and humanities that have broadened my thinking and sharpened my writing. Thank you to the members of the spring 2010 Global Health Faculty Research Seminar and to the members of the spring 2012 California Cultures Initiative, "CA Exceptionalism?: Conversations on Environment, Health and Risk," for helpful feedback and stimulating exchange. Thanks also to the smart graduate students in my spring 2012 seminar "The Cultural Politics of Dietary Health," for helping me to explore the limits of ideas that are central to this book.

The UC Multi Campus Research Program on Food and the Body (MRP) has been an incredibly rich source of intellectual energy and a vital source for feedback as the chapters of this book were coming together. I am grateful to the Office of the President for funding our cross-campus collaborative learning and exchange, and to all the faculty members and graduate students who have participated in our dissertation retreats, public events, and works-in-progress meetings, especially those who provided feedback on chapter 2 and chapter 4 (twice!). Mike Ziser generously commented on an early draft of the introduction. Special thanks to Alison Alkon, Carolyn de la Peña, Ryan Galt, Lisa Jacobson, Kimberly Nettles, and Erika Rappaport for pushing me in all the right ways. Working closely with Lissa Caldwell and Julie Guthman in the context of the MRP has profoundly enriched both my scholarship and my life as a scholar.

Funding and logistical support have come from several sources. A Cornell University College of Human Ecology Dean's Fellowship in the History of Home Economics along with the expertise of the research librarians and archivists at the Mann Library and the Division of Rare and Manuscript Collections were essential to the research for chapter 3. I received support from UC Davis through yearly faculty research grants, a summer salary research grant, a Humanities Institute fellowship, and a faculty development award. Graduate student assistants Sara Rebolloso McCullough and Stephanie Maroney provided impressively efficient, thorough, smart, and reliable research support.

While most of the arguments in this book are new, some of the ideas in chapter 3 were previously published in "The Terror Within: Obesity in Post 9/11 U.S. Life," *American Studies* 48, no. 3 (2007). Some of the ideas in chapters 1 and 6 were previously published in "Critical Nutrition Studies," in *Handbook of Food History*, edited by Jeffrey Pilcher (New York: Oxford University Press), 2012.

My editor at Duke University Press, Courtney Berger, is exactly the kind of smart and empathetic editor I had always hoped to have. Her instinctive grasp of my vision for this book instantly impressed me, and I am extremely grateful for her ongoing, expert support for that vision. I am also thankful for the feedback I received on the manuscript at two different stages from an anonymous reviewer who kindly but firmly pushed me to make this a much better book. The entire staff at the Press has been a joy to work with. My copyeditor, Patricia Mickelberry, deserves special thanks for her meticulous but subtle work.

Many friends and colleagues have provided critical infusions of insight, energy, perspective, and confidence at various points along the way. Thanks especially to Aaron Bobrow-Strain, Susana Bohme, Christina Cogdell, Helen De Michiel, Ari Y. Kelman, Kirsten Ostherr, Kyla Wazana Tompkins, and Marilyn Wann. Many friends and family members have been along for parts, or all, of this long, wild ride, and I want to thank them for helping to take care of me and my family so that we could all continue to thrive despite the many challenges that writing a book inevitably presents. Thank you Sini Anderson, Megan Bower, Laura Kurre, Wendy Lichtman, EE Miller, Judith Moman, Sara Seinberg, Colleen Stout, Amy Yunis, Maggie

Zaccara and Jami Zakem. Louis Hagler caught crucial errors at the proofreading stage. Heartfelt thanks to André Jackson and Tashi Lhamo for providing perfect care for my children. Carrie Peters has no idea how important she has been. My mother-in-law, Kaci Ferrero, has been equally generous with her time, energy, love, and enthusiasm. Kusia Hreshchyshyn and Sonya Sanchez have been an inexhaustible cheering squad, and together with Loren Passmore and Orville Jackson they have also been an essential source of all of the most important forms of sustenance for me and my family.

Carolyn de la Peña fits into many of the groups I have already mentioned. She is a UC Davis colleague, a Food and the Body MRP member, and a friend, but when it comes to debts of gratitude I owe she is in a class by herself. Carolyn saw potential in me I did not know I had and has continuously given me the opportunity and impetus to meet it. She has read every word of this manuscript, sometimes more than once, and provided the kind of pointed criticism that I imagine every writer wishes they could give themselves.

Stacia Biltekoff, my sister and my neighbor, has been a steady, loving, helpful presence. My parents, Cecile and Steven Biltekoff, waited eagerly but very patiently for this moment to finally arrive, and in the meantime they did everything they could to help it to come along. Their close, affectionate relationship with my children is a beautiful outgrowth of their generous willingness to help out.

My children, Saskia and Ruven Freedberg, have been born and raised alongside this book. Sometimes people think that I would have finished it sooner had I not also had them, but I doubt that I would have had the courage and tenacity to finish it at all without them. The strength of their commitment to everything they do, especially learning and growing, has been a vital source of inspiration, motivation, and delight throughout the process of bringing these ideas to paper and this book to publication. I met their father, Shawn Freedberg, a few days after I defended the proposal for my dissertation. We knew instantly that we would make our life together, but I don't think either of us had any idea that this project would be part of it for so long or that his steady assurance, generosity of spirit, and epic kindness would become so integral to my ability to complete this work. Shawn, thank you for teaching me how to be thankful and for giving me so much to be thankful for.

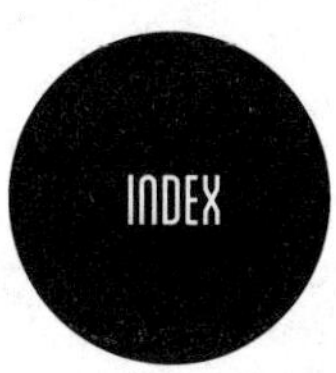

INDEX

Page numbers in italic type indicate illustrations.